# DEDICATION

This book is dedicated to all of the cancer patients for whom I have had the honor and privilege to provide care; to the residents, nurses, and all others who have helped me in this mission; and to my family who has supported me so that I may follow my passion to try to cure gastroesophageal and gastrointestinal cancer with surgery and to teach and inspire my students and residents to do the same.

# Table of Contents

# PREFACE

L earning you have cancer can be devastating. The initial diagnosis of cancer of the stomach or esophagus can leave you and your family in shock—changing your world in an instant. Finding your way through the maze of specialists and treatment options can be overwhelming. This book can give you information to put you on course to the best treatment plan for you and your cancer.

You are not alone. There are many who have been diagnosed and treated for these cancers before you, and many more will follow. Becoming educated about your disease is critical to participating in treatment choices and making informed decisions. The more you know, the more confident you can be that you are on the right course.

This book is part of a series of *Johns Hopkins Cancer Patient Guides* designed to educate newly diagnosed patients about their cancer diagnosis and the treatment that may lie ahead. The information provided will guide patients from the time cancer is confirmed to the completion of treatment. You do not necessarily need to read the entire book. Take your time, and review the chapters that are appropriate for you when you are ready. Resource information, including access to Johns Hopkins surgical oncologists, is also contained within these pages.

Don't feel the need to read the entire book at once. Rather, it is intended for you to read at your leisure and when you feel ready for additional information. It is not written to guide physicians in the treatment of stomach and esophagus cancer; it is written to guide patients.

Gastric (stomach) and esophageal cancer are considered together. The esophagus joins the stomach, and tumors of either have similar presentation, evaluation, and treatment plans. Both often present with eating problems and/or weight loss; both usually present at later stages, thus causing much lower cure rates than other cancers; and both are managed with multidisciplinary cancer teams with the mainstay of curative efforts centered on surgery. When referring to cancer of either the stomach or the esophagus, we use the term gastroesophageal cancer.

Until there is a cure or there are effective ways to prevent gastroesophageal cancer, the surgeons and oncologists at the Johns Hopkins Medical Institutions will continue to support patients who hear the words "you have gastric cancer" or "you have esophageal cancer."

We are here for you.

*Mark D. Duncan, MD, FACS*

# Introduction

# How to Use This Book
# to Your Benefit

**W**hen you have been diagnosed with cancer of the stomach or esophagus, you will receive a great deal of information from your healthcare team. You will also probably seek out some information on the Internet or in print. Friends and family members, meaning well, will offer you advice on what to do and when to do it, and will try to steer you in certain directions. Relax. Yes, you have heard words you wish you had never heard said about you—that you have cancer. Despite having heard that shocking phrase, you have time to make good decisions and empower yourself with accurate information so that you can participate in the decision making about your treatment.

This book is designed to guide you through the maze of treatment options and sometimes complicated schedules. It will help you put together a plan of action so that you can become a cancer survivor. While not all patients with esophageal or stomach cancer can be cured, many are, and your goal is to join that group. For those less fortunate, in whom the cancer is not cured, this book also offers strength and guidance.

The book is arranged into chapters and includes an index as well as credible resources listed for your further review and education. By empowering yourself with accurate, understandable information, you will be in a much better position to understand and participate more comfortably in the decision making about your treatment.

With the exception of only a few cases of esophageal or stomach cancer, you have the time to consider your treatment and to plan things well and confidently. Let's begin now with an understanding of what has happened and what the steps are to getting you well again.

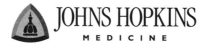

# First Steps—I've Been Diagnosed with Cancer of the Stomach or Esophagus

Finding out you have cancer of the stomach or esophagus can be an overwhelming experience. When patients hear the words "you have cancer," they are often left in shock. They may have trouble focusing on their feelings or understanding what they are being told. No one wants to have cancer. While everyone knows people, friends, or relatives who have had cancer, few think they themselves will. There are many immediate questions that come to mind: How did I get this? How long have I had it? Why don't I have pain or other symptoms? Why wasn't it detected earlier? I don't have a family history of this cancer, so how did I get it?

Cancer is more common than we realize. The American Cancer Society reports that one out of every three people in the United States will develop some type of cancer during their lifetime, and this does not include the common skin cancers. There are some cancers that tend to run in families, and family members may carry a genetic trait that predisposes them to cancer. These types include breast, ovarian, melanoma, and pancreatic cancer, as well as a small proportion of colorectal cancer. Cancers of the stomach and esophagus, however, are usually isolated in that the patient does not typically have a family history of these cancers.

While less common in the United States, cancer of the stomach, called gastric cancer, is the fourth-leading cancer in the world. The prevalence of cancer of the esophagus has been steadily increasing in the United States in the last decade. The esophagus is the muscular tube that connects the throat to the stomach. Cancers arise from the lining cells of the esophagus and stomach. More cancers are now being seen at the junction of the esophagus and the stomach. Symptoms of esophageal or gastric cancer include unintended weight loss, difficulty swallowing or eating, and anemia. The diagnosis is usually made endoscopically by introducing a flexible, lighted scope through the mouth into the esophagus and stomach. This procedure is called an *esophagogastroduodenoscopy*, or EGD for short. It is also called an *upper endoscopy*.

Risk factors have been identified for stomach and esophageal cancers. Gastroesophageal reflux (GERD) is a risk factor for esophageal cancer, although millions of Americans have reflux symptoms without developing cancer. Smoking and alcohol consumption are clear risk factors for one type of esophageal cancer. Hiatal hernia is a benign condition in which part of the stomach pushes up into the chest. This condition is common and is not a cancerous or precancerous condition.

Most cancers have no symptoms in their early course. It may take 2 years for a tumor to grow to the size of a pea. Prior to this time, cancer cells will be present, but are undetectable by current studies. Cancers of the stomach and esophagus usually are recognized when a patient develops symptoms of bleeding or obstruction. The earlier the cancer is detected and smaller it is, the easier it is to treat. Not every cancer can be seen by X-ray or imaging. Plain X-ray rarely detects cancers of the esophagus or stomach. Computed tomography (CT) scan or magnetic resonance imaging (MRI) can pick up tumors larger than 1 to 1.5 cm; however, these tests are not used to screen the general public. Performing an upper endoscopy can diagnose these tumors, but the relatively low frequency with which they occur does not support performing an endoscopy on all adults.

Once the diagnosis of gastric or esophageal cancer is established, there are two important questions that must be answered to guide treatment strategies:

- How extensive is the cancer within the esophagus and/or stomach?

- Has the cancer spread to lymph glands or other sites outside the esophagus and stomach?

The answers to these questions determine the stage of your cancer. The stage of your cancer determines your treatment options and prognosis for cure.

While all patients are concerned about how and when their cancer was diagnosed, the most important concern is the evaluation, management, and treatment once the diagnosis is made. That is what this book is for—to help guide you, the cancer patient, through the experience of cancer treatment. You will feel at times overwhelmed. The cancer itself affects your body and your health. The treatments you may need can also significantly affect your health. There often is more than one option in approaching the cancer or forming a treatment strategy. You will meet with cancer specialists from many medical and surgical fields. Even with support all around, you may feel alone.

You are not alone. Cancer is treated by a team, and each member of the team plays an important role, with you as the most important team member. There are many people who have had this same cancer, and you can find support groups through the hospital, the cancer center, your community, or the American Cancer Society.

### SELECTING YOUR ONCOLOGY TEAM

You want your cancer care to be provided by experts. This is not a simple health problem or a simple operation. This is cancer. Seek out a cancer center that is accredited by the Commission on Cancer for your care. Cancer centers employ professionals who specialize in the care of the cancer patient, including surgical oncologists, medical oncologists, radiation oncologists, pathologists, imaging radiologists, oncology nurses, and psychosocial support staff. These centers will provide genetic counseling for patients who need it. They will have regular cancer conferences or tumor boards to collectively review cancer patients in a multidisciplinary discussion. While there are many doctors who treat patients with cancer, you want your doctors to spend most or all of their time treating cancer. An accredited cancer center must meet standards of care and track all of its cancer patients, each year sending the data to the national cancer data bank.

In selecting the treatment center, you may wish to consider the following: What is the reputation of the center? Is it certified? If a cancer center has been certified by the American College of Surgeons Commission on Cancer, it has met or exceeded multiple standards for cancer care. Your doctor or others you know may also tell you about the reputation of the center. Does the center participate in clinical trials? You may not need or want to be in any trials, but the center should have resources so that information on trials is available to you. You will probably need both inpatient (hospital care) and outpatient treatment.

When you are meeting with a physician or surgeon, it is OK—in fact it is a good idea—to ask about his or her experience with cancer treatment. If you have been referred by your family doctor to a surgeon, ask questions such as:

- How many cancer operations do you do?
- What other type of operations do you do, and how much of your time is spent doing cancer treatments?
- Are you board certified? In what field?

- How long have you been in practice, and do you regularly attend the tumor board conference?

- Who are the other members of the team that I would be seeing, and what are their roles?

- How long will you follow me as a patient? (A gastric or esophageal cancer surgeon should follow you not just through the operation, but should have regular follow-up for the next 5 years.)

These are all questions you have the right to have answered before deciding if a physician or surgeon is right for you. You must be comfortable with this person's bedside manner. What about his or her approach to educating patients about treatment options or disclosing information? Your doctor should be empathetic and comfortable delivering both good and bad news.

Remember, you will be establishing a bond with your cancer doctors. You will be relying on them to provide the best care and to keep you informed about options and plans. You will be entrusting your health to them. Ask yourself when you meet a doctor if you want this person to command your ship in the fight against cancer.

It is not unusual for a patient or a physician to request a second opinion after an initial consultation. This may be particularly true if the patient has initially gone to a smaller or rural facility where oncology specialists may not be available. A second opinion is when you go to another cancer specialist or group to have them review your information and render an opinion. There may be many reasons for seeking a second opinion. You may not be comfortable with the doctor you have seen or the information you have been given. You may wish to see an expert who treats your condition more commonly. Distance, convenience, or expense may be issues. It can be reassuring to hear that different doctors in a different center agree with the plan outlined by your doctor. You may find that you are more comfortable with one doctor or center over another.

Remember that you are the most important member of your cancer treatment team. You are a unique person, and your particular care should be tailored to you. To play an active role during your therapy, you should become familiar with gastroesophageal cancer. You can do this by:

- Being involved in decisions that affect you

- Learning about your cancer and your treatments so you are confident you understand them

- Talking to your doctors and nurses about your worries or concerns

- Keeping your clinic and hospital appointments for your evaluation and treatment

- Knowing how to contact your cancer team for questions or issues that arise during the course of treatment

## GETTING RECORDS: BIOPSY, RADIOLOGY STUDIES, AND OTHER TESTS

Once you have been diagnosed with stomach or esophageal cancer, you should request copies of all tests that have been done, including all imaging studies (CT scan, X-ray, MRI, ultrasound), endoscopy reports, and pathology reports of biopsies. Be sure to obtain copies of your medical records. Indeed, you should begin your own folder or portfolio of your cancer records. This will help not only now but down the road so that you can always have a record of what treatment you have received. Continue to request copies as you continue your journey. No matter who sees you—surgeon, medical oncologist, or radiation oncologist—they will want to review these records.

They will also want to see the actual films or images and not just the written report from the facility where the imaging was done. You should contact the facility where the studies were done. They will provide either copies of the films or a CD with the images. You can then bring them to your first consultation with a new doctor or send them in advance. It is helpful to give the physician a chance to review your scans or films before having you waiting in the office. You may wonder why you need to gather these images if they have the reports. An accredited cancer center is required to review the images, and most importantly the pathology slides, to verify their accuracy. Upon re-review, a pathologist who specializes in gastroesophageal or gastrointestinal cancer may discover that an error was made or that the pathology was not interpreted the same as on the original report. What was called invasive cancer may only be precancerous changes, or vice versa. Accuracy and experience are key in pathological diagnosis. Your treatment plan depends on experienced review of all available data.

You should also bring records of your general medical health and condition, including current and prior diseases, medications, allergies, and operations. Not only will it help your cancer doctors understand you better, it will save you much time, considering that you will need to provide this information many times in the course of your treatment.

Most patients bring along a family member, loved one, or friend to their appointments at the cancer center. This helps so you don't feel quite as weighed down by other concerns regarding your treatment. Writing down questions in advance can be very helpful to ensure that all of your questions are addressed.

**LEARNING ABOUT YOUR DISEASE**

Cancer is a disease in which cells in the body grow out of control and keep dividing so that more cells are made. Cancer cells can directly invade into adjacent tissues or organs, or they can spread to distal areas in the body such as the liver or the lungs. A growth of cancer cells that is detectable is called a tumor. Cancer of the gastrointestinal tract, particularly cancer of the stomach or esophagus, becomes noticeable to the patient when it causes bleeding, obstruction, or weight loss. Not all patients have these symptoms. Many patients wonder why they don't have pain. In fact, most cancers are painless when they are first detected. The earlier a cancer is detected, the better the chance it can be cured.

When doctors evaluate cancers of the stomach and esophagus, they first try to diagnose whether a cancer is present and where it may be located. Then they want to know if there is any evidence that the cancer has spread. Looking at the cancer and looking for spread of cancer is called "staging." The earlier the stage, the better the chance of cure. Also, knowing the stage or extent of the cancer helps determine what the best specific treatment or treatment options are.

Let's consider each kind of cancer in turn. There are two primary types of esophageal cancer: squamous cell carcinoma and adenocarcinoma. The squamous cell cancers used to be the most common and are associated with older patients, those with a smoking history, and those with high alcohol consumption. They can occur anywhere along the esophagus. Adenocarcinomas of the esophagus, once rare, are now the most common type. Adenocarcinomas are associated with GERD and occur almost always at the lowest end of the esophagus right where it joins the stomach. The overwhelming majority of the millions of people who have acid reflux do not get cancer, but those who have changes in the esophagus seen by endoscopy, called *Barrett's esophagus*, have a much higher chance and have to be followed closely. Patients with Barrett's esophagus are followed by repeat endoscopy and biopsy. Those with early changes, called *low-grade dysplasia*, are followed by their gastroenterologist. When a biopsy demonstrates *high-grade dysplasia*, they may need surgery or more intense surveillance at a specific center with expertise in this condition. *Carcinoma* means invasive cancer.

Stomach cancer is usually adenocarcinoma. It can be subdivided into two distinct types. The intestinal variety of adenocarcinoma of the stomach is associated with increased age and occurs more often in men. The diffuse type occurs more often in women, tends to occur at a younger age, and can spread diffusely through the stomach wall. This adenocarcinoma is often called *signet ring* type because of a typical appearance of some cancer cells under the microscope. Risk factors for stomach cancer include gastric polyps, pernicious anemia, prior *Helicobacter pylori* infection (the bacteria associated with peptic ulcers), and prior stomach surgery in which part of the stomach was removed.

Another kind of cancer seen in the stomach is lymphoma. Lymphoma is a cancer of the lymph gland tissue, but it can appear as a stomach tumor. Gastric lymphoma is very different than usual gastric cancer, and the treatment is very different as well. Gastric lymphoma is often treated with just chemotherapy, whereas gastric adenocarcinoma needs surgery to be cured.

A final tumor seen in the stomach is the *GIST* type. GIST stands for **g**astro**i**ntestinal **s**tromal **t**umor. These tumors can be very large. About half of them are cancerous, but even looking under the microscope it can be hard to determine. GISTs are very different from the usual gastric cancer and will be discussed separately.

Most patients diagnosed with esophageal or stomach cancer are older, with ages typically ranging from 55 to 85 years. These cancers can be seen in younger patients in their 40s. Gastric cancer is seen far more commonly in people of Korean, Japanese, or Chinese descent.

Early cancers are limited to the superficial layers of the esophagus and stomach. More advanced tumors have deeper invasion into the wall of the esophagus or stomach. The spreading of cancer to sites outside of the original organ is called *metastasis*. Metastatic cancers can spread to

11

local and regional lymph nodes around the esophagus and stomach. More advanced spread is to lymph nodes in the neck or deep in the chest or abdomen. Distal spread of cancer through the bloodstream can occur to the liver, lung, or bone. Gastroesophageal cancers can also spread by directly invading the adjacent organs such as the liver, pancreas, or airways. Finally, there can be extensive spread along the inside of the abdominal cavity, called *carcinomatosis*. This cancer is not always picked up on preoperative CT imaging and may not be seen until surgery. Metastasis of cancer to distant organs and the presence of carcinomatosis are both ominous signs of cancer that cannot be cured.

When you enter the world of cancer, you will learn a whole new vocabulary. Initially this is overwhelming, but it is very helpful to begin to understand what you will be fighting even before the first visit. If you have done some homework, you will know the right questions to ask and be prepared to understand the answers given. You will also have time to begin considering what treatments are available or will likely be recommended. That is what this book is for.

## DIAGNOSIS AND PROGNOSIS

Initially, all the information on your medical reports and from your doctor will seem incomprehensible to you. It may sound like Greek. By the end of your treatment, however, you will be familiar with the information and will be quoting it yourself with confidence and knowledge. Many patients say they can write a book on their disease; it's probably true—indeed, some do.

Before your first visit, let's review what happens after a biopsy has been performed. The majority of biopsies are done at the time of an upper endoscopy when the gastrointestinal doctor inserts a scope through the mouth into the stomach. Any abnormal area or tumor is sampled with a small needle, and a small bit of tissue is removed and sent to a pathologist. It usually takes a few days to receive a final result. The small bit of tissue provides a tiny window into the big picture of gastroesophageal cancer that is to soon be uncovered. This piece of tissue provides information about the type of stomach or esophageal cancer you have and a few specifics about its characteristics. It does not tell more than this—how big the tumor is, how long it has been there, or whether or not it has spread. Other tests and/or surgery will give much more information, so it may be premature to ask the doctor too much about your prognosis, the exact stage of the disease, and precisely what the details of your treatment will be. Along with information from your imaging studies (CT scan, MRI, or endoscopic ultrasound), the biopsy information provides your doctor with what is needed to determine your treatment recommendations.

## TUMOR GRADE

In addition to diagnosing cancer or precancer changes in the tissue, the pathologist can also look at the degree to which the cells look normal or look aggressive, thus determining the *grade* of the cancer. It is better to have low-grade or *well-differentiated* cancer cells than high-grade or *poorly differentiated* cancer. In between is *moderately differentiated.*

There are additional tests of the cancer specimen that may be more commonly done when the entire tumor is removed at surgery. The information from the prognostic tests on the entire tumor rather than the tiny biopsied piece is preferred by the pathologist.

It can be easy to confuse stage with grade. This is a common mistake. However, they are quite different. Grade, as just discussed, is related to cell growth and is determined from the biopsy information. Stage, by contrast, requires more details about the cancer and its behavior and measurements.

## GASTRIC AND ESOPHAGEAL CANCER STAGING

When gastroesophageal cancer is diagnosed, it is crucial to evaluate the extent of the tumor and determine the presence or absence of metastasis. This is called staging. Stage combines several pieces of information about the primary tumor and spread to lymph nodes and any other organ involvement. It is closely tied to the prognosis. Generally speaking, the more advanced the stage, the more serious the cancer and the poorer the outcome. The staging system adopted in the United States utilizes the TNM system, which stands for tumor, nodes, and metastasis. First is the "T" which refers to the primary tumor in the stomach or esophagus. It indicates the size of the tumor and whether it has spread through the layers of the wall of the stomach or esophagus.

$T_x$–Cannot assess the size or depth of the primary tumor

$T_0$–The tumor is not detectable

$T_1$–Tumor limited to the mucosal lining

$T_2$–Tumor invades into the wall of the stomach or esophagus

$T_3$–Tumor invades through the wall

$T_4$–Tumor invades through the wall and into adjacent organs

The "N" tells whether there is evidence of spread of cancer cells to the lymph nodes.

$N_x$–Information not available or lymph nodes cannot be assessed

$N_0$–No spread to lymph nodes

$N_1$–Spread to 1–2 lymph nodes

$N_2$–Spread to 3–6 lymph nodes

$N_3$–Spread to 7 or more lymph nodes

Finally, the "M" refers to distant metastases—the presence or absence of cancer in organs or sites remote from the primary esophageal or stomach tumor.

$M_x$–Information not available or cannot assess

$M_0$–No distant spread

$M_1$–Spread to other areas including distant lymph nodes or organs such as liver, lung, or bones

The findings of T, N, and M taken together give the stage. Each distinct cancer (esophagus, stomach, breast, lung, colorectal, etc.) has a staging system, and the prognosis for each can be quite varied. Survival for gastric cancer and esophageal cancer, unfortunately, is not very good.

The biopsy can determine the cell type, whether there is invasion, and the grade of the cancer. Cancers can spread directly into adjacent tissue and can spread to other organs in the body. A CT scan (or MRI) is the best single test to evaluate spread. Cancer of the esophagus can spread to adjacent lymph nodes in the neck, chest, or abdomen or distally to the lung or the liver. Cancer of the stomach usually spreads to lymph nodes around the stomach and in the upper abdomen, and can go to the liver. Large lymph nodes can be seen by CT, MRI, or ultrasound. When tumors are removed at surgery, many smaller lymph nodes can also be examined. When cancer has spread to lymph nodes, there is a much greater chance that it has also spread elsewhere in the body.

## ESOPHAGEAL CANCER

*Stage 0* esophageal cancer is *noninvasive* cancer. It is also called high-grade dysplasia or carcinoma in situ. The cancer cells are limited to the lining of the esophagus and do not invade into any deeper layers.

*Stage I* esophageal cancer has invaded into the wall of the esophagus. The tumor is still small, and there is no spread of cancer detected in the lymph nodes or elsewhere in the body.

*Stage II* esophageal cancer invades into but not through the wall of the esophagus and has spread to lymph nodes or invades through the wall of the esophagus with spread to few lymph nodes.

*Stage III* esophageal cancer invades through the wall of the esophagus and/or includes the spread of cancer cells to more lymph nodes. This is locally advanced cancer.

*Stage IV* esophageal cancer is advanced cancer with spread to distant sites beyond the lymph nodes such as liver, lung, or bone. The presence of cancer in other organs is determined by scans and/or biopsies of the sites. Prognosis for cancer at this stage is very poor.

## GASTRIC CANCER

*Stage 0* gastric cancer is noninvasive cancer. It is also called high-grade dysplasia or carcinoma in situ. The cancer cells are limited to the lining of the stomach and do not invade into any deeper layers.

*Stage IA* gastric cancer has invaded into but not through the wall of the stomach, and there is no spread of cancer detected in lymph nodes or elsewhere in the body.

*Stage IB* gastric cancer is a small cancer that has invaded into but not through the wall of the stomach or has spread to few lymph nodes.

*Stage II* gastric cancer includes tumors that have invaded the full depth of the stomach wall without spreading to lymph nodes; or invaded to an intermediate depth and spread to few lymph nodes; or invaded to a limited, shallow depth and spread to more lymph nodes. There is no sign of spread elsewhere in the body.

*Stage III* gastric cancer has invaded more deeply with cancer cells spread to lymph nodes; or a large tumor has invaded through the stomach wall into surrounding organs without cancer cells having spread to lymph nodes. There is no sign of cancer elsewhere in the body.

*Stage IV* gastric cancer is advanced cancer with either spread to distal organs such as the liver, lung, brain, or bone. Prognosis for cancer at this stage is very poor.

There are two methods of cancer staging: clinical and pathological. Clinical staging is an estimate of the stage based on physical examination, X-ray, MRI and other imaging, and endoscopic findings. Pathological staging is more precise and is based on the pathological examination of tissue removed at surgery. This allows exact measurement, including depth of invasion, and detailed examination of all removed lymph nodes rather than relying on seeing "large" lymph nodes with imaging. The pathologist uses a microscope to see if cancer cells are in the lymph nodes and evaluates any other tissue samples that might have been obtained. Some treatment plans call for chemotherapy, radiation, or both before any surgery. In these cases, a clinical stage is used because the treatment will be given, or at least started, before the tissue is removed.

Your doctors determine your stage both to plan treatment and to give you a survival estimate—what is the chance you are or will be cured. This is a good time to point out, however, that you are not a statistic. You are a person. When a cancer doctor says someone has an 80% chance of cure, it does not mean the person is 80% cured. When it comes down to it, you either are cured or you aren't. Unfortunately, even with all of the information available, your doctors cannot immediately after treatment know if you are cured. If cancer is seen on tests or imaging, your doctors may be able to diagnose it. After treatment, not seeing cancer on any test or image is a good sign; but doctors cannot definitely say no cancer is present. Individual cancer cells are too small to detect with tests and X-ray scans or images. There is no test that proves someone doesn't have cancer. Rather, doctors rely on volumes of information about treatment and outcomes of thousands of patients with each type of cancer, and they use the staging information to group patients together. Thus, an 80% cure rate means that 8 out of 10 patients with this stage of this cancer are cured by the treatment, and 2 are not. At the time an estimate of cure is given to you based on your stage, you don't know where you individually will be in the statistic. The chances may be high (or low) that you will be cured, but neither you nor your doctors can know for certain which group you will be in. This uncertainty is part of what it means to be a cancer survivor. You survive, hoping to be cured, but with the knowledge that you might not be and that only time will tell. For better or for worse, you do not have to wait forever to know. In cancer of the stomach and esophagus, if there is no sign of cancer 5 years after treatment, you are cured. You are doing what is needed to be on the survival side.

## AN UNPLEASANT TRUTH

Unlike breast cancer, where 85% of patients are cured, and colorectal cancer, where 66% are cured, the majority of patients with esophageal and gastric cancer are currently not cured despite therapy. Do not despair, and do not give up hope—many still are cured. In the last decade, an increased number of patients with either gastric or esophageal cancer can be cured. As is true for most solid tumors, surgery is the mainstay of therapy. Of all patients with gastroesophageal cancer, however, the sobering fact is that only a quarter (25%) of stomach cancer and only 4% of esophageal cancer will be cured. The chances are much better if your studies do not show distant spread of the cancer and you are a surgical candidate. The 5-year survival or cure rate with surgery presently is around 35% for patients who have surgery with no evidence of remaining tumor at the end of the procedure. More recent data suggest that earlier detection will mean higher cure rates.

This honest reporting of the data is not meant to be demoralizing but to underscore the severity of the disease and balance this against the treatment options and the magnitude of the operations. Yet we are still optimistic and hopeful. As more of these cancers are detected at an earlier stage, and as we advance our knowledge and understanding of adding chemotherapy and radiation to surgery, we are able to offer cure to more patients with gastroesophageal cancer.

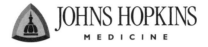

# CHAPTER 2

# MY TEAM—MEETING YOUR TREATMENT TEAM

The many medical professionals who make up your treatment team all share a common goal—for you to be well again. Each has a specific role to play, and the team members work together to coordinate your care. Here are the major members of your cancer team:

> *Surgical Oncologist.* This surgeon specializes in cancer surgery. He or she may be a thoracic surgeon or a general surgical oncologist. The surgeon performs operations to remove the cancer and surrounding lymph nodes. Often, the surgeon is the first specialist you see. The surgeon not only performs the operations but also directs the postoperative recovery and follow-up. The surgeon is often the one directing therapy in the early phase of your treatment

*Medical Oncologist.* This physician specializes in the systemic treatment of gastroesophageal cancer with chemotherapy and/or targeted therapy and overall management of cancer patients. The medical oncologist often is the main healthcare provider for people with cancer. In addition to medical treatment of cancer, the medical oncologist specializes in cancer follow-up, pain management, and, if needed, end-of-life or hospice care. The medical oncologist often coordinates care between cancer specialists, and often directs therapy in the later phases of your treatment.

*Radiation Oncologist.* This doctor specializes in treating cancers of the esophagus and stomach with radiation therapy. Not all patients will require or be considered for radiation treatment.

*Gastroenterologist.* This doctor is a gastrointestinal specialist who performs endoscopy to see the esophagus and stomach and to biopsy tissue for diagnosis.

*Radiologist.* This doctor interprets the X-rays and images and may perform biopsy procedures guided by images.

*Pathologist.* This doctor examines the microscope slides of your tumor to determine the diagnosis of cancer. The pathologist also evaluates all tissue removed at surgery to determine the size of the tumor, the depth of invasion, and whether the cancer has spread to lymph nodes. You will not likely meet the pathologist.

*Nurses.* You will meet many nurses in your journey through treatment. Oncology nurse practitioners work with physicians and surgeons and are often a part of the immediate team providing direct care. Nurses assist with chemotherapy, radiation, and, of course, all aspects of surgery and hospitalization.

*Social Worker.* This individual specializes in support as well as addressing financial, home, and transportation concerns you may have.

## MAKING YOUR INITIAL APPOINTMENT IN THE CANCER CENTER

You may have been referred to either a surgeon or an oncologist once the diagnosis of cancer has been made. The doctor or doctors who you will be meeting should be specialists in managing stomach or esophageal cancer. Many surgeons treat cancer patients, but for these specific tumors you are better off if this is an area of expertise for that surgeon. It has been well documented that patients have better outcomes for these more complex cancer operations if they are treated at high-volume centers or by surgeons who perform these operations more regularly. At a cancer center, the surgeon, oncologist, and radiation oncologist work together for patients. Depending on the type or stage of your cancer, you may be counseled for surgery, chemotherapy, radiation, or a combination of treatments.

When making the initial appointment, be sure that the person you are speaking with knows you are a new patient with a new diagnosis of cancer. We like to offer all new cancer patients an appointment within the week. If you have just been told you have cancer, you do not want to wait for an appointment, and you shouldn't have to. Most facilities do arrange for patient appointments quite promptly. It is estimated that it takes a few years for one of these cancers to grow to a detectable level. Thus, it is not an emergency to get to the cancer doctor; but for peace of mind and to "get things going" in your treatment, you should be seen promptly. This time frame also means that you have the necessary opportunity to make good decisions; you should not feel rushed into treatment at a facility or by a doctor with whom you are not comfortable. Make sure you place yourself in capable hands. You can get information on most centers and on the doctors at that center. Usually, this information is available online (see Chapter 11). You may look to see if there is a particular doctor you think you may prefer to see over another; or you may have heard of a specific doctor or had one recommended to you. You can request a specific surgeon or oncologist.

Be sure to get a specific address and clear directions as to where you are to go and what time you are to report there. Many physicians see patients at more than one location, so ask the scheduler to double-check which location you are to be seen at. If you haven't been to the facility before, leave yourself some extra time to get there. Ask about parking and the best way to get to the office from the parking area. Arriving early will help you feel more comfortable when you get there, rather than feeling rushed or flustered. It also gives you the time to sit in the waiting area, take a few deep breaths, and review your questions one more time. You want your visit to be productive so that when you leave you have a plan that has been explained and that you are comfortable with.

Ask the office assistant if your doctor often has much of a wait before being seen. While no one likes to be kept waiting, it is not necessarily a bad sign. Many times, the best doctors are frequently requested and are very busy. Each doctor should try to keep close to a schedule, but the most important concern is that the doctor takes the time necessary with you to fully evaluate your situation and to explain clearly the plans, tests, or treatment options and decisions. He or she should answer all of your questions in language you understand. A good visit with a reputable doctor often takes more time than is written on a schedule. While this level of care is to your advantage, you may have to wait a little longer. Remember, your doctor is working with other cancer patients and families who also have fears, concerns, and questions.

## WHAT TO BRING WITH YOU FOR THAT FIRST CONSULTATION

Most likely the person who helped schedule your appointment has gone through a list and advised you what to bring. In case this information was not clear, the following information will help to ensure that your visit is as productive and efficient for you (and your doctor) as possible.

Bring with you—or even better, send in advance—all X-ray, CT scan, and/or MRI images that have been done. Be sure to also have the reports of each study. Your doctor may not need to look at every X-ray you have had but will certainly want to personally look at some, if not all, of the tests. The doctor may have requested that the microscope slides of the pathology be shipped in advance so an expert at his or her center can review the slides and assess the interpretation and diagnosis. Also, you should know in advance if your insurance company requires pre-authorization for having additional tests. The doctor could find that the studies you have had done are incomplete or inadequate for treatment planning. When this occurs, the doctor may want to get additional imaging done while you are there for the visit or soon thereafter. The doctor may also request that you leave the images or copies with him or her so that they can be reviewed with a radiologist at the cancer center. Each doctor may have specific experts whom he or she trusts in evaluating images or slides. If you have any trouble obtaining your studies or reports, talk with the office of the cancer doctor you will be seeing. While this may be the first time you have had to navigate these waters, the cancer team has done it before and can help you through.

Bring reports from any endoscopy with pictures (color if possible). Objects in a black and white copy of a picture of the inside of the esophagus or stomach can be hard to see clearly. Usually, your doctor will want to look at the pictures with you and show you what is there. A good doctor will also show you on your X-rays what he or she is talking about in terms of the location of a tumor or any sign of spread. You should ask your doctor to review these images with you if he or she has not already done so.

If you have seen any other cancer doctors, surgeons, or specialists, you should bring copies of their evaluations and reports. Each doctor or center will come up with their own evaluation, but an outside report may contain information that will be helpful in determining the best care. If you have heart disease or any other significant medical condition that may affect your ability to have surgery or other treatment, you should have with you your most recent treatment or evaluation records related to that condition or disease. Many patients with heart disease successfully undergo major cancer surgery and treatment. Bring with you the names and office phone numbers of your doctors so that the cancer center doctors and surgeons can directly contact your physicians if needed.

## WHO TO BRING WITH YOU

Bring a trusted family member or friend with you to the visit. You will not remember all of the details of your discussions with the doctor. Again, it is easy to feel overwhelmed. When individuals are stressed, they often only retain a fraction of the information that is conveyed to them. The doctor will likely be talking a great deal, presenting a large amount of information. It is all familiar to the doctor, but it may all be new to you. It is hard to keep it all straight in your mind. The person who comes with you can help make sure you get the information and get it recorded. This will be very helpful when later discussing the recommendations with other family or friends.

## WHAT ELSE TO BRING

Be sure to bring an accurate list of your medical conditions, operations you have previously had, medications (including vitamins and herbs) you are taking, and allergies. It is important to know if anyone in your family has had cancer and what type. If you have had prior surgery, try to know exactly what was done. This information is particularly important for any prior gastrointestinal, abdominal, or chest surgery.

As you can see, there can be a large amount of material to assemble. Put together a folder or binder containing your cancer-related and health information. It will be very helpful to you not just at the beginning but throughout your cancer care. Keeping everything together will ensure that you and any doctor you see will have access to your information. The easiest time to start this collection is at the beginning. It can include any notes you make or any information given to you by the doctor or center. It can also include lists of your questions and the answers to them.

## WHAT QUESTIONS TO ASK DURING YOUR VISIT

Preparing in advance a list of questions to ask will make your visit with your doctor as efficient and optimal as possible. Often your doctor will already address these concerns, but you can make sure each gets answered. The following list is written for a visit to the cancer surgeon, but it may be adapted to an initial visit with the medical oncologist as well. Specific questions about the surgery or radiation treatment will be covered later.

- What type of cancer do I have?

- Did you find anything new based on your examination or evaluation?

- What stage of disease do you think I have based on the current information?

- Do I need further tests or studies to determine my stage or treatment?

- Did your pathology team review and confirm the accuracy of my biopsy results?

- Am I a candidate for surgery? How did you make this determination?

- What surgery would you recommend or do you perform for my cancer?

- Is gastric or esophageal surgery an area of your expertise?

- How soon will my surgery be scheduled?

- Should my cancer be treated by surgery, chemotherapy, or radiation? Or all three?

- Should I have chemotherapy and radiation first followed by surgery, or surgery first?

- Do you anticipate that I will need chemotherapy? Why (or why not)?

- Do you anticipate that I will need radiation treatment? Why (or why not)?

- Who else will be involved in my care, and what are their roles?

- When should I see the medical oncologist or other cancer specialists?

- Who will be my contact person for questions?

- Who will be coordinating my care?

- Do you have a patient navigator?

- How are my subsequent appointments scheduled?

## WHAT ADDITIONAL TESTS ARE NEEDED

For patients diagnosed with gastric or esophageal cancer, the staging evaluation needs to be complete prior to making treatment decisions. Usually an upper endoscopy (scope) has already been done to diagnose the cancer. If a CT scan has not been done, it should be performed to assess the extent of tumor invasion or spread of cancer. The combination of endoscopy, biopsy, and CT scan usually gives enough information to make a treatment plan. Endoscopic ultrasound can be used to try to get more accurate information on depth of tumor invasion and may be used to biopsy lymph nodes. Not all cancers require this procedure, and its use is particularly uncommon in stomach cancer. In esophageal cancer, the better staging information of endoscopic ultrasound can be useful in choosing between surgery up-front or chemotherapy and radiation. Endoscopic ultrasound is an outpatient procedure that uses a scope with an ultrasound probe on the tip. A positron emission tomography (PET) scan or PET/CT scan may be requested to further evaluate any potential spread of cancer to distal sites.

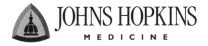

# CHAPTER 3

## TAKING ACTION—
## COMPREHENSIVE TREATMENT
## CONSIDERATIONS

Treatment for esophageal or gastric cancer considers all possible options: surgery, chemotherapy, and radiation. For surgery of the esophagus, the initial staging will determine if you are a candidate for potentially curative treatment (not stage IV). If your staging already shows you cannot be cured, then surgery is not an option. Chemotherapy or chemotherapy with radiation may be offered to slow the disease progression, to try to improve your ability to eat, and to maintain your quality of life as best as possible. This approach may also apply if your health is so poor that you are not a candidate for any surgery.

For potentially curable cancer of the esophagus, the main choice is between surgery first or chemotherapy and radiation first (or without surgery). Traditionally, surgery was thought necessary for cure. Now it is recognized that a small number of people with cancer of the esophagus can be cured by the combination of chemotherapy plus radiation without having surgery. This approach is called *definitive chemoradiation therapy*. Most patients have a better chance of cure if surgery is added. When chemotherapy and radiation come first and surgery follows, it is called *neoadjuvant therapy*. Surgery is usually 5–6 weeks after the last dose of radiation. When surgery comes first and chemotherapy and radiation follow, it is called *adjuvant therapy*. Chemotherapy, when started after surgery, does not usually begin for 4–8 weeks after the day of surgery. It is not currently clear if one sequence offers a better chance of survival than the other. Some patients with cancer will be offered surgery up-front or alone without chemotherapy, depending on both the stage of the cancer and the health, comorbidity, or frailty of the patient.

Similar choices exist for gastric cancer—surgery up-front, followed by possible chemotherapy or chemotherapy and radiation, depending on the findings at surgery; or chemotherapy and radiation first, followed by surgery. Chemotherapy plus radiation without surgery is not considered curative treatment for gastric cancer.

Each cancer center may have its own preference. Your doctors should discuss all of these options with you and explain why they recommend a given treatment. The major considerations of each of these treatments are discussed in this chapter.

## SURGERY

Surgery is recommended for all patients with gastric or esophageal cancer who are medically fit and potentially curable (stage I to III disease). Surgery of the stomach or esophagus is serious business. These procedures are more complicated and can have more profound effects on the body than most other abdominal or cardiac operations. Not all of the details discussed here may pertain to you. Make sure you talk with your surgeon to ask specifically what type of operation is proposed, what the risks are, what the expected recovery is, and what you can expect after surgery.

The goal of surgery is to remove the tumor and surrounding tissue, including lymph nodes next to or near the cancer, and then to reconstruct the gastrointestinal tract so that you can resume eating. Surgery has risks right up-front, but most people recover quite well. Removal of the esophagus or part or all of the stomach does permanently affect your eating. Patients are advised about the *postgastrectomy* diet, which basically is eating smaller meals more frequently. In stomach or esophagus surgery, the remaining intestines when put together will not have the same amount of reservoir space to take a very large meal. Fortunately, most people are able to eat reasonably well after recovering from surgery. Indeed, for many it was the inability to eat that brought the cancer to a doctor's attention.

### ESOPHAGECTOMY

The esophagus is the muscular tube that connects the throat to the stomach. Removal of the esophagus is a serious operation and should be performed at a major hospital center. The operation can be performed either through the chest or through the abdomen and the neck. The choice of technique depends most on the training and preferences of the surgeon. There is no uniform agreement among cancer centers as to which is better. Each accomplishes the same plan—to remove the esophagus with the cancer and to replace the gap with part of the intestines, usually the stomach. The chance of cure with either approach appears to be the same. Almost all esophageal surgery in the United States uses one of the following two methods.

### Transthoracic Esophagectomy

In this approach, the surgeon opens the abdomen and the right side of the chest through two separate incisions to directly remove the esophagus. It is often called the Ivor Lewis procedure. The stomach is then brought to the upper part of the chest and sewn to the remaining top portion of the esophagus. A chest tube will be placed to drain fluid out of the chest following the operation. This tube is usually left for several days and removed at the bedside when the amount of fluid draining is less than 100 cc per day.

Some centers offer a minimally invasive version of the transthoracic esophagectomy called *minimally invasive esophagectomy*. In this approach, multiple smaller incisions are used with special instruments and video equipment to view the procedure. If offered, make sure the surgeon has considerable experience in this type of procedure.

**Transhiatal Esophagectomy**

In this approach, the surgeon opens the abdomen and the left side of the neck through two separate incisions to remove the esophagus. The stomach is then pulled up to the neck just above the breastbone and reconnected to the top part of the esophagus. There is no incision in the chest and usually no chest tube. The hiatus is an opening in the diaphragm between the chest and the abdomen. This operation stretches that opening to remove the esophagus without needing to open the chest.

## GASTRECTOMY

*Partial* or *distal gastrectomy* involves removal of the distal two-thirds of the stomach with all of the adjacent fatty tissue and lymph nodes. The small intestine is then sewn back to the upper portion of the stomach. Cancers of the distal stomach are treated with distal gastrectomy. Most of the stomach still needs to be taken because the surgeon must divide tissue at least 6 cm (over 2 inches) in each direction on the stomach from the visible tumor to ensure total removal of the cancer. The edge where the tissue is divided is called the *margin*. One of the main goals of cancer surgery is to get negative margins. This means no cancer cells spread to the margin.

*Total gastrectomy* means removal of the entire stomach and adjacent fatty tissue and lymph nodes. The small intestine is then brought up to the lowest portion of the esophagus just at the top of the abdomen and sewn together. The intestine may be doubled back on itself to create a small pouch. Tumors of the middle or upper stomach require total gastrectomy to achieve the 6-cm margin.

Tumors at the junction of the esophagus and stomach are often treated as tumors of the lower esophagus and can be managed by resection of esophagus and part of the stomach.

## STAGING LAPAROSCOPY

In some cases of esophageal or gastric cancer, a surgeon uses a minimally invasive surgical procedure to evaluate the abdomen before definitive therapy is performed. In this procedure, the surgeon inserts a scope into the abdomen to examine the cancer and search for spread. This can be helpful in borderline cases where the possibility of cure is in doubt. If indicated, a feeding tube can be placed at the same time.

## CHEMOTHERAPY

Chemotherapy is the use of medications to treat cancer. There are many different cancer drugs, and they are not all alike. Many patients are afraid of the idea of chemotherapy or think that it makes everyone sick or makes everyone's hair fall out. You may have had friends or relatives who had chemotherapy. Before jumping to any conclusions, realize that the many different "chemo" drugs have different risks and different side effects. While they may cause fatigue, illness, or even serious problems, most people do reasonably well with chemotherapy.

Systemic chemotherapy is delivered through the blood-stream, targeting cancer cells throughout the body. The goal of chemotherapy is to destroy cancer cells outside the field of surgery or those remaining after surgery, to slow the tumor's growth, or to reduce side effects. Although some chemotherapy can be given orally, most drugs used to treat esophageal or gastric cancer are given intravenously. One of the common drugs used for gastroesophageal cancer is Adrucil (5-fluorouracil), also called 5-FU. This drug is usually given as a continuous intravenous infusion, but there is one version that can be taken as a pill, although it may not be appropriate for your cancer or treatment plan. Other chemotherapy drugs include Platino (cisplatinum), Eloxatin (oxaliplatin), VePesid (etoposide), Camptosart (irinotecan), Adriamycin (doxorubicin), and Taxol (paclitaxel). When you meet with the medical oncologist, he or she will discuss the specific medications recommended, the schedule with which they are given (such as once a week, or one week per month), and the length of treatment or number of treatment cycles. Chemotherapy often extends over months. Drugs are commonly given in combination, so you may be receiving more than one drug at the same time. Traditionally, chemotherapy has been considered after surgery; and this remains the standard treatment at most centers.

## NEOADJUVANT CHEMOTHERAPY

One consideration for either gastric or esophageal cancer is to give chemotherapy prior to undergoing planned surgery as the first phase of treatment. This is usually combined with radiation. In such cases, it is referred to as neoadjuvant therapy. This option is also within the standard of care. The mission of chemotherapy in either case is both to treat areas of the body beyond where the surgeon can reach and to treat the tumor and local lymph nodes. Chemotherapy and radiation are given to hopefully shrink the tumor, thus increasing the chance of surgery getting completely around the tumor—that is, achieving negative margins. Giving chemotherapy before surgery also increases the number of patients who get chemotherapy, since not all people recovering from surgery are able to or feel up to undergoing chemotherapy. Sometimes, chemotherapy and/or radiation are given first in patients who may not be surgical candidates or whose tumor looks like it may not be removable. After the neoadjuvant therapy, the patient is reevaluated for response to the treatment and reconsidered for surgery. In many cases, a patient receiving chemotherapy and radiation as initial treatment may need nutritional support with a temporary feeding tube. This is because the side effects of the chemotherapy and radiation treatment make it difficult for patients who have already experienced substantial weight loss to take in adequate nutrition and regain their lost strength.

CHEMOTHERAPY GIVEN AFTER SURGERY

If you have had surgery as the main treatment or initial treatment, the final pathology report together with the operative findings will determine your pathological stage. The medical oncologist will then determine if chemotherapy is a good idea based on all of this information. Stage 0 cancer certainly needs no chemotherapy, and early Stage I cancer may not benefit much from chemotherapy. Patients with Stage II and III cancers of the stomach and esophagus are usually offered chemotherapy to increase the chance of cure above that which is gained by surgery alone. In this setting, the chemotherapy is called adjuvant treatment because it is given as an adjunct. In patients with advanced, incurable cancer, chemotherapy may be recommended not because it may cure the disease, but to try to slow it down or prevent or limit problems. This is called *palliative chemotherapy.*

DEFINITIVE CHEMORADIATION THERAPY

When chemotherapy plus radiation is given as the only treatment, with no surgery, it is termed *definitive chemoradiation.* In esophageal cancer, there can be some long-term survivors or cures without surgery, but the chance of cure appears to be substantially lower. Still, this option exists for those patients who may not be medically fit to undergo surgery.

If you are deciding whether to take chemotherapy before or after surgery, many factors come into play. You have to ask your doctors what they think the chance of cure is without any further therapy. How much can the chemotherapy increase the chance of cure? By 3%? By 5%? By 15%? The numbers may only be somewhere in this range; in other words, chemotherapy may, indeed, increase the cure rate for gastric and esophageal cancer, but not by a lot. Or ask your doctor, what are the expected or usual side effects, and how does my overall condition affect my ability to tolerate treatment? Age, too, is a factor in deciding for whom chemotherapy is appropriate. Elderly, frail patients, for example, may be advised that chemotherapy would not be wise for them. Someone young, say in their 40s or 50s, would probably be advised to take chemotherapy as part of the treatment plan.

Stage of the disease, grade of the cells, and other clinical and pathological factors influence this decision-making process. There is no "one right answer" that serves everyone. Even cancer doctors, when asked about taking chemotherapy if it offered a 5% benefit, do not agree if they would take it themselves. Some would, some would not.

How much you worry can also influence this decision. If you were told that the survival benefit of taking chemotherapy is only increased by 3%, would you want it, or would that be too low a number to make it worth the potential problems or risk? Or, if you were told that the chance the chemotherapy would improve your chance of cure is only 1%, would you do so because you would take any little help? Younger patients, particularly if they have children in the home, will usually undertake chemotherapy even if the chance of benefit is low. In general, older patients with grown families and with more medical problems may want to see a higher probability of benefit before deciding to "put up" with chemotherapy.

SIDE EFFECTS OF CHEMOTHERAPY

Chemotherapy, a form of systemic treatment, can cause a second wave of distress. Symptoms include fatigue, gastrointestinal problems (particularly diarrhea), and rarely hair loss (unlike breast cancer treatments in which hair loss is common). Anticancer drugs usually go after rapidly growing cells, which include cancer cells and normally rapid-growth cells such as the lining of the intestine, the hair, and the bone marrow. Steps can be taken to treat or reduce possible side effects of chemotherapy. Today, not everyone experiences side effects. Medications are available to treat or reduce nausea. Continued activity, therapy, or exercise have been shown to reduce the side effects of fatigue. Chemotherapy is usually administered intravenously and given on an outpatient basis. Most treatments last 3–6 months.

## FOCUS ON THE POSITIVES

A good outlook is to focus on what chemotherapy is designed to do to help you. The drugs are going after cancer cells that have spread elsewhere in the body. You can use visual imagery to picture how these drugs work, and focus on those images. Remember, you are trying to climb the survival curve by taking chemotherapy.

Most patients feel well the day of the treatment. If side effects are to occur, they most commonly happen the night following chemotherapy or the next day. It is important to realize that some patients will react differently to chemotherapy than will others. Talking with other patients can help tremendously in facing this "battle," but it will not inform you of how you personally are going to feel and what side effects, if any, you may experience.

You want the advice of the medical oncologist in deciding which drug(s) will be right for you. Generally, the oncologist will have a specific recommendation based on the type and stage of your cancer.

PRECAUTIONS DURING CHEMOTHERAPY

During your course of chemotherapy, your blood will be sampled at designated intervals to make sure your red blood cells and white blood cells are staying within normal limits. It is common for cancer patients to be anemic. If either of your blood counts is too low, your doctor might decide to give you special medicines to boost your blood counts to a normal range.

Be aware of people around you who have a cold or the flu because your immune system is being taxed during the chemotherapy process. Small children especially may have bacteria or germs that may be harder for you to fight off when on chemotherapy.

How much chemotherapy impacts your life depends as much on your age, overall health, and recovery from surgery as it does on the chemotherapy. Some people who are still working are able to continue to do so despite chemotherapy. Usually, you can keep up daily routines at home. Remember, there is a beginning and an end to chemotherapy. The side effects are easier to deal with when you know they are for a limited time.

**RADIATION**

Radiation is not used on its own in treatment plans for cancers of the esophagus and stomach, but it is often used in conjunction with chemotherapy and surgery.

Radiation is the exposure of tissue to ionizing radiation that can kill rapidly growing cells. Radiation can shrink tumors and can help kill cancer cells in adjacent lymph nodes. In doing so, it helps achieve what is called *local control* of the cancer, which usually means a decreased chance of cancer coming back in the same area. Often, radiation is given together with chemotherapy. The chemotherapy usually increases the effect of the radiation. Unlike chemotherapy, the damage done to normal tissue by radiation is generally permanent, and it adds up. Once an area of the body has reached its limit of radiation, no further radiation can be given to that area. There have been vast improvements in radiation therapy as a local treatment over the last decade or so. Special technology is used so that only the tissue that needs to be irradiated is irradiated. The radiation oncologist maps out the area of the body to receive radiation, thus minimizing the dose to surrounding tissue. Although there is some risk to radiation side effects for the heart and lung tissue, this risk is markedly less today than it was years ago. Radiation may make the overlying skin a little pink, resembling mild sunburn (another type of radiation). There may be tenderness. Treatment is usually daily, Monday through Friday, for 5–6 weeks. Although this means going every day to the radiation facility, you are in and out quickly, usually in less than half an hour.

Radiation does not hurt. It feels the same as getting a chest X-ray, which means you feel nothing at all. However, the effects of radiation are cumulative—they add up. That is why you may start getting fatigued toward the last few weeks of treatment. Maintaining your activity level, even just walking regularly, has been shown to reduce this side effect. The chest or upper abdomen area is exposed during radiation therapy treatments, but you are behind closed doors with just your treatment team looking in on you.

Before radiation begins, special measurements of you will be made to ensure that the radiation beams are lined up exactly the same way to irradiate the same area consistently and precisely. This process is called *simulation*. A few tiny tattoo marks (little blue dots) will be made on the skin as part of the preparation process. These dots are usually permanent. Some people proudly show off their surgical scars; you can also be proud of these tiny tattoos.

Just as there are clinical trials for chemotherapy, there are also trials in which radiation treatment is done differently than the conventional external beam radiation. You should ask your radiation oncologist whether there are any trials for which you might be a candidate.

## OTHER TREATMENT CONSIDERATIONS

### CLINICAL TRIALS

New and innovative treatments are developed by doing clinical trials. Most current cancer treatments are the result of previous clinical trials. Without clinical trials, doctors could not improve the treatment of gastroesophageal cancer, nor could ways be developed to try to prevent it in the future. They are the cornerstone and forefront of the science of cancer treatment today. Your doctors may at any given time during your treatment discuss with you opportunities to participate in a clinical trial. You should be open-minded. Hear what is being offered as part of a study.

Clinical trials are research studies in which people agree to try new therapies under careful supervision to help doctors identify the best treatments with the fewest side effects. These studies help improve the overall standard of care for the future. Clinical trials may offer you an edge over standard treatment, offering you access to methods that may actually define treatment for people diagnosed with gastric or esophageal cancer in the future.

There are many different kinds of clinical trials. They range from studies focusing on ways to prevent, detect, diagnose, treat, and control cancer to studies that address quality-of-life issues that affect the patient. Most clinical trials are designated a particular phase depending on the goals of the trial. Each phase is designed to learn different information, and each builds upon information previously discovered. Patients may be eligible for studies in different phases depending on their stage of disease and therapies anticipated, as well as treatment they have already had. All patients are monitored at specific intervals while participating in any study.

## GASTRIC LYMPHOMA

Gastric lymphoma is a cancer of the lymph cells found in the stomach. It is quite different from most gastric cancer, and like other lymphomas, it is treated primarily with multidrug chemotherapy and possibly radiation. A less common variation of gastric lymphoma is MALT-lymphoma, which is associated with stomach infection with *Helicobacter pylori* organisms. MALT-lymphoma may be better considered as a precancerous condition; interestingly it can often be treated successfully with antibiotic treatment targeted at *H. pylori*. Surgery is not commonly required for gastric lymphoma.

GASTROINTESTINAL STROMAL TUMORS (GISTs)

GISTs are a special type of stomach cancer that is very different from the other types. GISTs can occur anywhere in the gastrointestinal tract. The pathologist can easily diagnose GISTs both by appearance under the microscope and because they carry a specific marker called c-kit, which can be detected with special stains. Unusual about GISTs is that the pathologist often cannot distinguish a malignant (cancerous) tumor from a benign one. This uncertainty is why we use the word *tumor* rather than trying to say which one is cancerous. About half of stomach GISTs are malignant. GISTs can grow and invade into the organs surrounding the stomach including the pancreas, liver, colon, or diaphragm.

GISTs are managed primarily by surgery. After removing the tumor, your doctors may recommend taking a novel chemotherapy medicine called Gleevec (imatinib). This newer drug is specifically targeted to the mutation found in GISTs, and taking Gleevec appears to decrease the chance of recurrent tumor or prolong the interval before recurrence. This medicine is not like traditional chemotherapy drugs. It is taken as a pill once a day and has few severe side effects. Many patients do have some symptoms of gastrointestinal upset, but this is usually manageable. Gleevec is also used for patients with metastatic or recurrent GIST. The response to Gleevec can be dramatic.

# CHAPTER 4

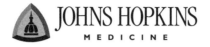

# BE PREPARED—THE SIDE
# EFFECTS OF TREATMENT

### RECOVERING FROM SURGERY IN THE HOSPITAL

Gastrectomy and esophagectomy are major procedures. Esophagectomy often takes 5–6 hours, and can take even longer. All patients will go to the surgical intensive care unit the night of surgery. On average, esophageal surgery patients stay between 1o and 14 days in the hospital. Gastric surgery has a shorter recovery but is still often a week in the hospital. There are very real risks with these operations, and each different surgical approach tries to minimize these risks while removing the tumor and surrounding lymph nodes. Chest or abdominal surgery is painful, and patients receive narcotic pain medicines to help manage the pain. The first 2 days are the worst, and thereafter the pain and discomfort get better each day. Do not be shy about asking for pain medications. Patients do not get addicted to narcotics due to use for postoperative pain, which follows a predictable pattern. Usually, patients are given a patient-controlled analgesia (PCA) where they can hit a button to give themselves small doses of narcotic pain medicine every 6 minutes. This usually works better than pain shots every 3–4 hours. Most patients are not given liquid to drink or food to eat for 4–5 days after surgery (a little earlier with stomach surgery). Before patients begin drinking water again, they undergo an X-ray in which they swallow contrast dye to ensure there is no leak.

There are several things your doctor and treatment team will do to help your recovery and to try to decrease the risks associated with surgery. They will instruct you on how to use an incentive spirometer, a small plastic device that measures how big a breath you are able to take. After surgery, especially with an abdominal or chest incision, it hurts to take a big or deep breath. But it is important to breathe deeply, otherwise fluid can build up in the tiny air sacs in the lung and cause fever or lead to pneumonia. As with most disease or complications, it is better to prevent the problem than to have to treat it. Pneumonia is one of the biggest risks after this operation. You should use the spirometer (which is easy) for several minutes every hour you are awake while in the hospital.

Another risk is the development of blood clots. Blood clots form in the veins, usually in the legs or in areas where blood pools. Blood clots cause swelling in the legs and can break off and go to the lung, which is much more dangerous. Everyone retains some fluid after surgery, so leg swelling is common. Your doctor will monitor for blood clots after surgery. The risk factors include surgery, immobility, cancer, and age. Clearly, any patient with gastric or esophageal cancer is at a higher risk for forming blood clots. There are three main ways to combat them. You will usually be given a small dose of a blood thinner. This small amount, typically given as a shot just beneath the skin, has been proven to decrease the risk of blood clots. It does not significantly increase the risk for bleeding. It is a very important part of your care. In addition, you will have special stockings with inflatable plastic wraps around your lower legs. These wraps periodically inflate and deflate, in effect giving your legs a massage. These pneumatic stockings have also been proven to decrease the risk of blood clots. They should be used while you are in the hospital bed recovering from surgery. You do not generally need to continue the pneumatic stockings or the blood thinner after leaving the hospital unless specifically directed to by your physician. The other important thing is to get up and walk. Walking frequently helps the blood circulation and decreases the risk of clotting. All of these approaches decrease the risk of blood clots but do not totally eliminate it.

These operations are a big deal, and there is risk involved. With operations of this magnitude, there is the chance that a patient may not recover to leave the hospital. While no one wants to talk about the possibility of death, with this type of cancer and these types of treatments, it has to be discussed. In cancer centers that treat esophageal cancer, the risk of dying in the hospital following surgery is about 4% or less. This is in comparison to a risk of up to 1o% at hospitals or centers that rarely perform esophageal surgery.

The biggest risk has to do with lung complications, leaks, or infection. A leak refers to the failure to heal at the site where the stomach is reconnected to the upper esophagus. Infection can occur at the surgical site below the skin or in the chest or abdomen. Patients can also develop irregular heart rhythms that may need treatment. Because of the size or scope of these operations, almost half of all patients have some type of complication, although many may be relatively minor. Despite these risks, because of the severity of the disease, surgery is still the mainstay of curative treatment.

Because patients often have had significant weight loss, nutritional support is commonly used to help them through treatment and recovery. This may include placement of a feeding tube either before or during surgery. When a tumor is blocking the esophagus, it is difficult to get adequate nutrition through. A feeding tube can allow nutrition while under treatment. A *G-tube* is a feeding tube directly into the stomach. A *J-tube* goes into the small intestine (jejunum). Everything about this disease and treatment can make it hard to eat. Chemotherapy and/ or radiation can take away patients' appetite. In the initial period after surgery, most people do not eat much, even when the diet is advanced and unrestricted. It is typical to lose 10–15 pounds in the weeks following surgery, and some people lose even more. Fortunately, almost everyone stabilizes. Nutrition can also be given intravenously. This is called TPN for total parenteral nutrition. Getting nutrition into the intestine is better and has fewer complications than nutrition through the vein.

Most patients when discharged from the hospital can eat, walk, shower, and use the bathroom. Usually all tubes, intravenous lines, and so forth have been removed, although some patients may still be getting nutritional support from a feeding tube if they required it before surgery. There may be stitches or staples still in the skin, which will usually be removed at the first postoperative visit with the surgeon.

## WOUND INFECTION

The most common complication after any gastrointestinal surgery, including surgery of the esophagus and stomach, is an infection at the surgical site. Infection occurs because the tissue is exposed to bacteria from the gut when the stomach or esophagus is open during the time of surgery. Antibiotics are administered prior to the start of the operation; this reduces but does not eliminate the risk of infection. Half of all surgical wound infections appear after the patient has left the hospital. Signs of wound infection include fever, chills, redness of the wound that may spread, increased tenderness or swelling that was not present before surgery, and any purulent drainage of fluid from the incision. Indeed, after hospital discharge, any drainage of fluid should be reported. Wound infections are managed by opening the skin to drain the infection. Antibiotics are often not required unless there is significant cellulitis (infection into the tissue surrounding the wound). Saline-moistened gauze or a similarly treated gauze sponge is used to lightly pack the area and is then changed once to three times daily, depending on the wound and the treatment plan. If the wound has to be opened, it may take weeks or even months to fully heal. A newer technique that accelerates wound healing is the wound vacuum system. In this technique, foam is sealed to the skin and connected to a backpack-style vacuum device that draws fluid and drainage away from the wound. The "wound-vac" is typically only changed 2–3 times per week.

## UNEXPECTED SURGICAL FINDINGS

Sometimes, when a surgeon opens a patient to perform a cancer operation, he or she finds much more spread of cancer than was seen from tests and scans before surgery. In this case, it may not make sense to remove the stomach or esophagus if the cancer is very advanced and survival appears to be short. If cancer of the esophagus has spread to the liver, it cannot be cured. Unfortunately, there is no benefit to trying to remove the spread of cancer, and if it has already gone to the liver, then taking out the esophagus does help the patient live longer or have less symptoms. If esophageal cancer is Stage IV, then the procedure is halted and the esophagus (with the cancer) is left intact after performing a biopsy to be certain of spread. While you would like to have the cancerous organ "out," in this circumstance it doesn't help.

Stomach cancer spread to the liver may not be curable, but patients may live for a considerable time, maybe even years. With stomach cancer, it is still better to get the stomach tumor "out," even with limited spread to the liver. Left behind, stomach tumors can bleed or obstruct.

## LONG-TERM SIDE EFFECTS OF SURGERY

Esophagectomy and gastrectomy each significantly alter the ability to eat. While most patients recover sufficiently, some specific problems can occur. Up to one-third of patients undergoing esophagectomy can have difficulty swallowing long after surgery due to narrowing or stricture at the site where the stomach was sewn to the upper esophagus. This problem is recognized by increasing difficulty swallowing or inability to eat solid food. Strictures are both diagnosed and managed by endoscopy. The narrow area is gently stretched to a greater width, which sometimes requires a few sessions to be effective. Patients can also have a sensation of early satiety (feeling full after having eaten little). The stomach pulled up in the chest can have delayed emptying. Patients who have had their stomach removed need vitamin $B_{12}$ replacement lifelong. Gastrectomy patients can also have flushing and/or sweating associated with cramping discomfort after eating. This is termed "dumping syndrome" and is due to rapid entrance of food into the small intestine. It usually resolves without treatment over time.

Talk with your doctor if you are experiencing any symptoms related to difficulty eating. There may be specific recommendations for your diet based on the operation you had and the symptoms you are experiencing. All hospitals have nutritionists on staff, and you should meet with the nutritionist after recovering from surgery to discuss your dietary needs and ways to help manage any symptoms you might have.

## SIDE EFFECTS OF CHEMOTHERAPY

There are various side effects to chemotherapy that a patient may experience while undergoing treatment for gastric or esophageal cancer. Some are easily controlled, and some may be more difficult. Not all patients have the same response to chemotherapy, and you may have few significant side effects. The following are the more common potential side effects that you should discuss with your oncologist. Understanding these possibilities ahead of time will help you prepare for what might happen and cope with what does happen.

### NAUSEA AND VOMITING

This side effect is relatively common with many forms of chemotherapy drugs. Fortunately, there are now newer antinausea medicines (called antiemetics) that have significantly reduced the incidence or severity of nausea and vomiting. Any pain medicine you are taking may also contribute to nausea. If nausea and vomiting is severe, resulting in the inability to keep down liquids, dehydration can result, and patients may need to be admitted to the hospital for intravenous rehydration. You may be able to make some changes in your eating and drinking to help manage nausea. Such changes include:

• Eat a light meal before chemotherapy.

• Eat smaller amounts of food and liquid at one time.

• Eat bland foods and liquids.

• Maintain hydration with liquids between meals.

- Drink mostly clear liquids (e.g., water, apple juice, herbal tea).

- Eat saltine or dry crackers when feeling nauseated.

- Eat cool foods or foods at room temperature.

- Avoid fatty, greasy, fried, or spicy foods.

- Avoid alcohol and caffeine.

- Suck on peppermint candies.

Ask your oncologist if you need an antiemetic medicine. You may wish to take this before chemotherapy treatment to prevent or reduce nausea. These medications include drugs such as Zofran (ondansetron), Kytril (granisetron), Compazine (prochlorperazine), Tigan (trimethobenzamide), Phenergan (promethazine), and Emend (aprepitant).

FATIGUE

Feeling exhausted or extremely tired is probably the most common side effect patients report. Fatigue is often a symptom of cancer and is certainly frequently encountered during treatment. Certainly surgery is a cause of fatigue, and healing and recovery can take months. The surgeon may say, "pain gets better first, and then appetite returns, but what takes the longest is your energy level." Surgery can knock you down hard, but usually the fatigue experienced after surgery declines and energy levels steadily rise, with noticeable improvement each week. Chemotherapy and radiation, however, tend to cause fatigue in waves based on the timing of therapy. When radiation and chemotherapy are added after surgery, fatigue can be overwhelming in the first months. Fatigue from radiation is usually experienced by the third week of treatment and may continue for up to 6 months after completion of treatment. Fatigue from chemotherapy may fluctuate, with a pattern of tiredness accompanying administration of the drugs followed by recovery, or the fatigue may be constant until treatment is completed. In either case, it may feel like you are constantly tired, and this lack of energy may persist for up to a year.

Medical problems common in patients undergoing chemotherapy may also contribute to fatigue. These include anemia, dehydration from nausea or vomiting, and malnutrition. Particularly for patients with gastroesophageal cancer or those recovering from gastrectomy or esophagectomy, poor dietary intake due in part to the inability to eat large meals makes it hard to recover energy. Lack of sleep can deplete energy. Depression is another major factor that interferes with recovery of energy and activity levels.

If you are recovering from cancer and cancer treatment, you should try to maintain your daily routine as closely as possible. Being able to keep up with your daily routine can reduce the chronic feeling of fatigue. Activity, of course, promotes your circulation and prevents your muscles from weakening. Discuss with your doctor or nurse your fatigue level. Addressing your fatigue should be a part of your treatment plan.

NEUROLOGICAL PROBLEMS

One possible side effect of chemotherapy drugs commonly used in gastric and esophageal cancer is *peripheral neuropathy* (damage to peripheral nerves). The most common effect is damage to sensory nerves, causing numbness and tingling in the hands and feet. Less common are symptoms from motor nerves, which control voluntary movements. Symptoms of peripheral neuropathy include:

- Numbness, tingling, or burning in the fingers and/or toes, often described as a "pins and needles" sensation

- Difficulty writing, holding a cup, or buttoning a shirt

- Decreased sensation of hot and cold

- Muscle weakness

If you develop any symptoms of peripheral neuropathy, tell your doctor. Your doctor may prescribe specific medications that may help with some of these symptoms. Such medicines include Neurontin (gabapentin), Tegretol (carbamazepine), Lyrica (pregabalin), and vitamin $B_{12}$.

### DIARRHEA

Diarrhea is common with the chemotherapy agents used for gastric and esophageal cancer and with radiation treatment. Diarrhea is defined as more than two loose bowel movements per day. Diarrhea may also result from the use of antibiotics or from infection. If the diarrhea is severe, patients may need treatment either with intravenous rehydration or specific antibiotic therapy if they have infection. One type of infectious diarrhea is called *Clostridium difficile* colitis. It can occur when bad *C. difficile* bacteria multiply in the colon after prior antibiotic treatment decreases other bacteria. Signs of infection include fever, watery bowel movements, or stool that contains mucus or blood. Inform your doctor or nurse if you experience more than two loose stools a day for more than two days.

INFECTION

Cancer patients undergoing chemotherapy are at higher risk of developing infection because the treatment can weaken the immune system. Infections can occur in the gastrointestinal tract, lungs, urinary tract, or at any surgical site or wound. Signs that an infection has occurred can include fever, chills or sweating, a sore throat or mouth, pain or burning with urination, diarrhea, shortness of breath, a productive cough, swelling, and redness or pain around an incision or wound. Taking measures to reduce the risk of infection is particularly important between 7 and 14 days after each chemotherapy treatment. Wash your hands frequently; brush your teeth regularly; avoid large crowds and crowded rooms; and wash, prepare, and cook your meals thoroughly. If you have chills, take your temperature. Contact your doctor or nurse if you have a temperature of 101.5°F or higher. A fever or infection has greater significance when your immune system is weakened, and your doctor or nurse may need to evaluate you to determine if you need any antibiotic treatment or if you need to be admitted to the hospital.

MOUTH SORES

This condition is also known as *mucositis*. It is an inflammation of the inside of the mouth and throat and can result in painful ulcers. Keep your mouth clean and moist to prevent infection. Brush your teeth with a soft-bristled toothbrush and rinse regularly. Medications such as steroids can increase the risk of developing infection in your mouth. Avoid mouthwashes that contain alcohol, which can irritate the mouth. If you wear dentures, make sure they fit properly.

## HAIR LOSS

This side effect is less common in patients treated with chemotherapy for gastric and esophageal cancer than chemotherapy used for other cancers. Nonetheless, hair loss, termed *alopecia*, can be distressing because of the immediate impact on body image and one's sense-image. Hair loss, if it occurs, usually begins 2–3 weeks following the start of chemotherapy. The hair begins to thin or falls out in patches or strands. No treatment has been proven effective in preventing hair loss. Fortunately, hair regrowth usually begins 4–6 weeks after chemotherapy is completed.

The emotional impact of hair loss is underappreciated. It can be psychologically and physically difficult to cope with hair loss. Special programs, such as Look Good . . . Feel Better, are available free of charge at most cancer centers and show patients how to wear scarves or makeup to reduce the obvious appearance of hair loss. Ask your doctor if hair loss is anticipated in your treatment. If it is, you may wish to be proactive and take charge of your hair loss rather than wait for it to happen. Getting hair cut short can be a good advance move.

## ANEMIA

Anemia is very common in cancer patients, particularly those with gastric and esophageal cancer. Most patients are already anemic because of slow, minute blood loss from ulcerated tumors in the lining of the esophagus or stomach.

There is always some blood loss from surgery. This amount may be small or it may be significant requiring transfusion. Anemia can also occur as a result of chemotherapy or radiation due to toxicity to the blood-producing cells of the bone marrow. The red blood cells (RBCs) contain hemoglobin and carry oxygen to the tissue in the body. When RBC levels are low, the tissue may not receive adequate oxygen to work and function properly. In extreme cases, inadequate oxygen delivery to the tissue risks damage or death of tissue. Most people with anemia generally report feeling tired constantly or tiring easily. The fatigue that accompanies anemia can seriously affect a person's quality of life. Other symptoms of anemia include light-headedness, dizziness, or shortness of breath.

If you experience any of these symptoms, contact your doctor. There are medications available that can help replenish the RBC population, including Epogen or Procrit (epoetin alfa) or Aranesp (darbepoetin alfa). These drugs are administered with a small injection under the skin the same way some patients give themselves insulin. If your blood counts are dangerously low, your doctor might recommend a blood transfusion. He or she will discuss this with you. While the risk of transmitting a serious infection such as hepatitis or HIV is extremely low, and usually much less than the risks to your health of symptomatic anemia, the decision to transfuse blood is not taken lightly and balances all of the risks and benefits of the treatment.

## LOW PLATELETS

Platelets are the elements in the blood that help with blood clotting. When platelet counts are low, a condition called *thrombocytopenia*, patients are at risk for easy bruising, excessive bleeding after minor trauma or procedures, or even spontaneous bleeding. Chemotherapy and radiation are common causes of low platelet counts. The fall in platelets is generally seen 1–2 weeks after treatment, and it may take a month or more for counts to return to normal after the treatment.

## CHANGES IN MENTAL FUNCTIONING

Patients who are receiving chemotherapy as part of their treatment can have trouble with memory (remembering names, place, and events), concentration, and language. This condition has been referred to as *chemo brain*. Changes in memory, concentration, and language can occur up to 2 years after chemotherapy has been completed. These changes are often distressing. Notify your doctor of any such change. If you find that these symptoms are severe and affect your ability to function well, there are several things you can do. Make frequent lists to help plan and organize your daily activities. You can mark off each item as it is done. Keep essential items such as your keys, eyeglasses, and medications in the same place so they are easier to find. Enlist family and friends to help keep you organized, especially if you are taking multiple medications. After chemotherapy is completed, these symptoms usually subside with time. Bear in mind that some people who have not undergone chemotherapy report having these same symptoms. Many other factors can affect concentration and memory, including stress, anxiety, depression, and other medications.

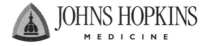

# CHAPTER 5

# STRAIGHT TALK—
# COMMUNICATION WITH
# FAMILY, FRIENDS, AND
# COWORKERS

C ancer is hard to deal with alone. Although talking about your cancer can be hard at first, most patients find that being honest and open about their cancer and the problems that arise helps them to handle their disease.

When individuals are diagnosed with cancer, it affects not only them and their family, but also friends, coworkers, and others. Who will you tell about your cancer? How much will you tell them—and when? Your treatment is likely to change their lives and routines as well as your own. Your cancer diagnosis and treatment will have an emotional impact on them, too.

Dealing with cancer is complex. It is often hard to communicate to close family and friends what is happening to you or how you are coping. Most people find it awkward, embarrassing, or even painful to discuss their illness. This can be true for your friends and family as well. After hearing that you have cancer, many people will want to ask you about your treatment plans. They may wonder whether, where, or when you will have surgery, or chemotherapy, or radiation. It is OK to answer them as best you can, but keep in mind that "I don't know right now" or "I haven't had the chance to make my plans yet" are also good answers.

Generally, discussing fears or concerns can put them into perspective. Although it may be hard to do so, discussing how you are coping with your diagnosis will make it easier to work with your family and friends and make plans for the future. You may have friends or family members who want to offer you advice or tell you to "cheer up" when you tell them about your sadness or fears. It is fine to ask them gently if they would be willing just to listen, without judgment or advice. You may want to say calmly, "Thank you so much for your concern, but I need to focus on something else today." Remember, this is your illness, and it is your decision whether you choose to discuss it.

**SHARING YOUR CANCER DIAGNOSIS**

You will go through many emotions as you consider your cancer and your treatment decisions. Only you can decide when to talk to your friends and family about having cancer. Most people need and want to talk to someone. Telling those close to them sometimes helps them begin to take in the reality of their situation, which otherwise can seem overwhelming. You should consider how much you want to share about your diagnosis. You may want to explain what cancer you have and which treatments you might need. You do not have to share your prognosis with everyone; however, most patients find it easier if at least their close family understands the seriousness of the cancer. You may even want to make a list of people who you want to tell about your cancer. People are very sobered by the news that someone has cancer. Think about what topics are too sensitive for you to talk about yet. Plan a response that is acceptable to you if these topics come up, and once you have shared what you wish to share, be prepared to politely end or change the conversation.

## TALKING WITH CHILDREN ABOUT CANCER

How and when to tell children that their parent has cancer is a difficult decision. Undoubtedly, your children will realize that something different is going on. It is always best to be honest. Even if we don't realize, children often overhear or become aware of important issues, and keeping the truth from them may well make them more scared than comforted. Explain in clear terms how treatment will fight the cancer. It is usually helpful to have both parents discuss this together. You may wish to tell your children soon after hearing the diagnosis, or you may wish to wait until after meeting with your doctors and deciding on a treatment plan. It is important to remember that the treatments for gastric and esophageal cancer have a major impact on you and will require a considerable amount of your time (as well as your energy). It helps to prepare your children or grandchildren for your illness.

Younger children are very dependent on their parents and are quick to notice stress or tension in the home. Despite their age, they will feel the stress. Cancer is often an unfamiliar concept to them, but it is important to talk with them about your illness. Do not overwhelm them with too much information. They tend to understand concrete ideas and make broad generalizations; yet how they react to upsetting news depends a lot on how the adults are handling it. You can let them know that you are very sick and that the doctors are going to work very hard to make you better. Your young children may worry that you are going to go away like other relatives who have passed on. Though you may not be able to reassure them that this will not happen to you, it is important to acknowledge their fears. Children may also irrationally believe your illness is caused by something they did. You need to reassure them that cancer is not their fault and not your fault. Illness is a part of life. They may also worry about catching cancer as if it were a communicable disease. Even if they do not voice this, you should reassure them that they cannot catch cancer from you. Let them know that it is OK to feel sad and that they should talk with you any time they are feeling sad. Try to maintain family routines as much as possible.

Older children may be anxious or even angry about how your cancer will impact them. Teenagers often view the world as revolving around them and may resent the changes in their lives. These responses are natural and can be magnified by the fear of losing a parent. You will have to decide how much to tell them, and when. Of course, each child is different, and each has his or her own experiences with illness or even death. Many children equate cancer with death, and it is important to acknowledge this possibility while emphasizing that the hope and goal of treatment is to cure you. Ask your children what they know about cancer and provide them with details they can understand. As you have undoubtedly already learned, your children know much more than you realize. Reassure them honestly about your treatment and prognosis. Teens may be particularly resentful when asked to help around the house. They have difficulty coping with the responsibility of partially filling a parent's role during times of upheaval. They may also feel guilty about their own resentment. Talk to your children about their feelings and about the role they play in the family. Communication is critical because your children face the upcoming challenge with you. You may wish to consider ways the teenager can contribute while still maintaining as much routine and typical parent–child boundaries as possible. Explain how you may need extra help for a while, but also take steps to show balance between family responsibilities and a normal teenage lifestyle.

## TELLING OTHER FAMILY MEMBERS

Telling other family members you have cancer can also be difficult. Parents, brothers, and sisters may wish to help. Families can be critical for providing and coordinating assistance during illness and treatment. Be prepared to accept offers of assistance. There can be unique family relationships and family dynamics that need to be considered. Remember, families often can and usually do come together during times of illness. This is a disease that affects the entire family. The feelings of fear and apprehension that you have are shared by your family.

## INFORMING YOUR FRIENDS

Just as with your family, it can be difficult to decide what to tell friends or coworkers. Whom should you tell? How much? When? It is usually best to be honest with the people closest to you. Keeping your cancer diagnosis a secret can cause you more stress at a time when you could use the support of others. Before you talk to others about your illness, think through your own feelings and your expectations of them. Often, people do not know what to say, which makes them feel awkward and uncomfortable. They may feel that it is easier to say little or nothing because they are afraid of saying the wrong thing. They may withdraw or distance themselves. Some may become overly considerate or intrusive. Most likely, your friends will want to help you, but they may be uncertain of how. Many people tell their colleagues or more distant friends only the basic information—that is, the type of cancer they have and the planned treatment. Information about stage, prognosis, symptoms, or body changes is often considered more personal. You may choose to share any of this information, particularly with those who are close to you or offer support, or you may choose to keep much of it, or all of it, private. This is your personal business, and whatever feels right for you probably is right for you. As with your family, offers of assistance are typically genuine, and it is beneficial for you as well as the helpers to involve them as needed.

## WHAT TO TELL YOUR BOSS OR COWORKERS

Whether to tell your coworkers about your illness is a very personal decision. You will need time off from work for your treatment, so it is advantageous to let key people know. You may choose to tell only your supervisor or closest associates, or you may decide to be very public about your situation. Many people are worried about how their disease or the time off required for treatment will affect their work or their ability to maintain their job. Fortunately, you have some job protection from the Americans with Disabilities Act (ADA). You should be able to work with your employer or boss on a schedule that will meet your medical needs. You are NOT required to tell your supervisor that you have cancer. It is fine to just explain that you are under doctor's care that will require you to miss time from work. Most people, however, choose to tell their boss that they have been diagnosed with cancer and that they will be undergoing whatever treatments are recommended. This is usually easier. Although you may choose to, you are not responsible for providing your employer with information about your prognosis.

### KEEPING FRIENDS AND FAMILY UPDATED

During and after treatment, the need or desire to update people on your situation can be a job in and of itself. You may wish to assign one person as the contact person to provide information on how you are doing, what treatments you are having, etc. This is true both during the initial evaluation when you may be undergoing several tests and during and following surgery, chemotherapy, or later follow-up. While updating people has usually been done with direct contact or phone, more recently people have also used a number of online resources to post information. Online sites are usually free, can be personalized, and can serve as a website to keep friends and family informed during difficult times. Some websites include a journal, a photo gallery, and a guest book. This can be a great way to communicate. Email is another way to keep friends and family updated without having to repeat the same message many times. It can be a great time saver to reduce the burden that communication can become.

## RECRUITING SUPPORT FROM FAMILY AND FRIENDS

People will undoubtedly ask what they can do to help you. Among the many things they can do are drive you to appointments, drive your children to school or events, run errands, make meals or deliver food, babysit, and help with housework. Remember that these people sincerely want to do something to help. Think what you would do in their place. While it can be difficult to accept help from others, it gives them an opportunity to help you and lets you focus on more important things related to your treatment. Some friends and family members will seem distant. This does not mean they don't care. Often, people can be uncomfortable with the notion of cancer and may avoid calling you or seeing you. They just don't know what to say. If individuals important to you seem distant, call them. Reassure them that you are still the same person. Remind them that cancer is just a disease, and laugh with them that it is not contagious. Remember that support from others is an important part of your treatment plan for you and for your family.

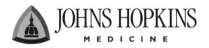

# CHAPTER 6

# MAINTAINING BALANCE—WORK AND LIFE DURING TREATMENT

Having cancer is a life-changing and, for many, lifelong event. The moment you are told you have cancer will likely be a time of deep emotional crisis and distress. In fact, most people say they have never faced a bigger or more frightening challenge. Fortunately, a diagnosis of gastric or esophageal cancer does not mean that your life comes to a halt, although it may feel that way. It will require some adjustments to your life, but you should continue to be as active as you have been, provided there are no medical reasons not to do so. Overall, you and your family should try to maintain life so that it is as normal for you as possible while you are having your treatment.

It may be difficult during treatment and care to ask for and accept help from others. Cancer treatment will alter roles in the family, play havoc with schedules, and create additional stresses for you and your family. Disruptions are inevitable but can be manageable. It is important for you and your family to talk about your schedules and about how treatment needs will impact them. You may need to design a new schedule to best meet your needs and those of your family with as little change as possible. This is also a good time to ask for help from other family members, friends, and neighbors. After all, one day they may need your help in a very similar way. Try to maintain routines as much as possible.

**MANAGING DAY-TO-DAY MATTERS**

MONEY

Dealing with cancer can reduce your family's spending money or savings. Medical care is expensive, and it can be hard to predict what your medical expenses will be. You and your family will need to learn more about your health insurance coverage. If you are unable to work due to illness or treatment, you will need to know how this will impact your income. Someone else in the family may need to get a job to help cover expenses.

LIVING ARRANGEMENTS

As you adjust to cancer, treatment, and illness, you may need more help and support at home than you have in the past. Accepting help can be hard because you may feel that you are losing your independence. This may also come at a time in your life when you or your family were already facing or at least discussing what living arrangements would be needed for you or your spouse as you age. You may need some home health care such as a visiting nurse, physical therapy, or other medical treatments. You may have to move in with another family member or have a family member move in with you during treatment. If you have to be away from home for all or part of your treatment, you should take a few personal effects with you. This way there will be something familiar even in a strange place.

## DAILY ACTIVITIES

During the course of your treatment, whether following surgery or while receiving chemotherapy or radiation treatment, you may need help with routine activities. This includes preparing meals, driving, cleaning, or even bathing. During chemotherapy, you should organize a calendar for when your treatments will be so that you can plan accordingly. You may want someone to accompany you for your treatments; this way the day can be a relaxed one for you, and someone else can manage or worry about getting you there and back, or handle any issue that comes up. Asking others to do things for you can be hard, but it is not a sign of weakness. As much as you are able, continue to carry out the regular household activities or leisure activities that you enjoy. Think about hiring someone or finding a volunteer through cancer support groups in your community or in your church. Remember, you are helping others when you allow them to help you.

## MANAGING THE SIDE EFFECTS OF TREATMENT

### PREPARING FOR SURGERY

In preparation for surgery, you will want to know how long you are expected to be in the hospital. You will want to know about activity, work, or driving after surgery. Ask about diet and weight change expected after surgery. Most patients lose significant weight after gastrectomy or esophagectomy.

## PREPARING FOR CHEMOTHERAPY

If you are scheduled to have chemotherapy, make a chart of when your treatments will be. Arrange for someone to go with you for chemotherapy treatments. You will be in the chemotherapy infusion center for several hours, so plan accordingly. Make sure you eat something before getting your treatment, as you need to maintain body weight to fuel your recovery. You may wish to bring a light meal or snack to your therapy sessions. Usually, if you are going to have gastrointestinal side effects, they will happen 12–48 hours after the infusion of chemotherapy. Request anti-nausea medications before treatment if you have suffered nausea as a side effect.

## PREPARING FOR RADIATION

This treatment is daily; most radiation facilities have patients in and out in less than 30 minutes. You may spend more time parking than actually receiving your treatment. Anticipate feeling fine until about the last 2 weeks of treatment. At this point, the cumulative effect of the doses may be causing increased fatigue. Give yourself extra time to rest at night. You may even want to take naps in the middle of the day. Consider which of your activities are the highest priority, and do the most important ones first to conserve energy.

## EATING DURING THERAPY

It is very common during treatment for gastric and esophageal cancer to have difficulty eating. As noted before, this can be due to the cancer or to any of the treatment modalities (surgery, chemotherapy, or radiation). Do not be hard on yourself if side effects make it hard to eat. Try consuming small, more frequent meals. Be sure to drink plenty of water or liquids each day. Let your doctor or nurse know of any side effects of treatment so they can prescribe medications to help with nausea and vomiting or diarrhea. Appetite loss is often the first side effect, characterized by a general sensation of not being hungry, getting full faster than normal, or feeling overwhelmed by a normal portion of food. While a reduced appetite may seem harmless, it can lead to severe weight loss, dehydration, fatigue, poor immune function, and malnutrition. Make every effort to eat as much as possible, as your nutritional needs are higher than before when undergoing cancer treatment. Cancer greatly increases the number of calories required on a daily basis, and the body may consume 1000 or more extra calories daily to build new healthy cells and successfully fight your cancer. Your oncologist may prescribe an appetite stimulant to increase your hunger. Appetite stimulants are usually reserved for people who have lost more than 10% of their body weight or are at risk for malnutrition. Not all appetite stimulants work for all patients, and they may take weeks to be effective.

Here are some suggestions to increase your ability to get nutrition if you are having trouble eating:

- Eat small portions throughout the day. Do not worry about eating regular meals; just try to eat small bites.

- Set a timer to remind yourself to eat. When you are not hungry, it is easy to allow 6 or 8 hours to pass without eating or drinking anything. You can set a kitchen timer to 1 or 2 hours and eat a few bites or drink when it goes off. This can be repeated during your waking hours.

- Keep food where you can see it. Place healthy snacks, bowls of peanuts, small candies, or dried fruit around the house, and eat one or two pieces when you walk by.

- Sip on beverages with calories. Hot chocolate, sports drinks, and fruit juices are great ways to help get in calories during the day. Keep juice boxes handy.

- Add nutritional supplements. Supplements such as Ensure, Boost, or Carnation Instant Breakfast provide a good source of calories, protein, and carbohydrates.

- Eat your favorite foods. This is no time to worry about fat or cholesterol. If it appeals to you, eat it.

OVERCOMING FATIGUE

The fatigue experienced by cancer patients is more than just being tired. It can be an overpowering sense of exhaustion that is not always relieved by rest. It can be mild, resulting in less energy to do the things you want, or it can be severe, affecting many areas of life and resulting in the inability to do basic activities. Fatigue can decrease both appetite and the energy to prepare meals, thus compounding the concern of adequate nutritional intake. Poor diet leads to more fatigue, and the vicious cycle continues. The best advice for combating fatigue is to try to eat a balanced diet including protein-rich foods such as meat, eggs, cheese, peas, and beans, and to drink 8–1o glasses of fluids a day. Preventing malnutrition and dehydration can help keep baseline energy levels up and provide the body with the fuel it needs.

## KNOWING WHEN TO ASK FOR HELP

There are certain signs that you might need help from your cancer care team. Talk to your doctor, nurse, or social worker if you have any concerns that seem too big to manage on your own or if any of the following occurs:

- You feel overwhelmed, depressed, sad, hopeless, discouraged, or empty almost every day or have lost interest or pleasure in activities that were once enjoyable.

- You notice extreme changes in your eating habits (eating too much or too little) or experience weight loss or weight gain.

- You have changes in your sleep pattern such as inability to sleep, waking too early, or sleeping too much.

- You find that others notice that you are slowed down or exhausted almost daily.

- You have trouble concentrating, remembering, or making decisions.

- You have thoughts of death (not just fear of dying) or suicide.

- You notice wide mood swings, from depression to periods of agitation or high energy.

Cancer treatment may cause some of these symptoms, but if these symptoms last for 2 weeks or longer or are severe enough to continue to interfere with your normal functions, you may need an evaluation by a mental health professional.

## CONTINUING WORK

Many patients are able to continue work while receiving chemotherapy or radiation treatment. Time missed from work can be minimal if planned relatively well. You may wish to continue working, as the stopping of work that occurs with treatment can add to your stresses. It may help your attitude to feel productive, be surrounded by friends and coworkers, and not spend every waking moment thinking about the cancer. There may be days that you work only half the day because of your treatment. If you are working and receiving radiation, you may wish to schedule your radiation early in the morning or late in the day. Be prepared for the side effects of your treatment, and give yourself extra time to rest as needed. A review of Chapter 4 will help you anticipate the possible side effects of your treatment regimen.

## STAYING HEALTHY DURING TREATMENT

During chemotherapy, you may be more susceptible to certain diseases, particularly if your white blood cells

(WBCs) go down in response to having received chemo-therapy. These are the days you are more vulnerable to get-ting a cold, flu, or other infection. If your WBCs are low, you should avoid the presence of young children because they can carry germs without appearing sick. Wearing a mask may be beneficial if you can't avoid children. Eating a balanced diet helps your overall health, including your immune system. Wash your hands frequently. It is advis-able to get a flu shot, but you should do so before starting chemotherapy. This is true for dental work, as well. You should have any dental work or teeth cleaning, if needed, completed before you start chemotherapy. If you need to travel by air while undergoing chemotherapy, wear a mask to reduce your risk of exposure to airborne germs. Your mission is to be healthy during your chemotherapy treat-ments and to reduce your exposure to infection as much as possible. Your blood will be periodically drawn to assess how your body's immune system is responding to the che-motherapy treatments.

## FINDING MORE TIME

Most people find it hard to fit everything into their family's schedule, even before the demands of cancer and cancer treatment. Consider the following tips for finding more time for yourself and your family:

- Take advantage of free or low-cost delivery services. Many grocery stores offer online shopping and home delivery. Several items can be delivered to your home, including prescriptions, DVDs, stamps, or dry cleaning.

- Spend less time in the kitchen. Take advantage of nutritious prepared and frozen foods readily available. Simple meals such as sandwiches can substitute for a more elaborate dinner.

- Do not try to clean the whole house. Concentrate on what matters most to you, like having the dishes washed or laundry done. You might hire a cleaning service or college student to do a more complete cleaning once or twice a month.

- Reconsider your family's schedule. Your loved ones may need to pick their more important or favored activities and take a break from some others.

- Rearrange your own activities and focus on one or two that are really important to you.

Cancer and cancer treatment is tough on a physical, emotional, and practical level. With all of the demands on your time, it can be easy to forget to make time for yourself. Decide which tasks are priorities for you and which tasks you can ask someone else to do or just leave undone. Setting aside time to do something you enjoy or just to relax and rest is an important part of the healing and recovery process. When you take care of yourself, you will have more of the energy and patience needed to fight your disease.

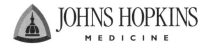

# CHAPTER 7

# Surviving Cancer of the Stomach or Esophagus— Reengaging in Mind and Body Health After Treatment

There comes a time when chemotherapy and radiotherapy treatments end and surgical scars heal. As a patient you may look forward to this time when you can begin to work toward returning to your life as it was before cancer. Some patients feel as if they have completed a long and difficult battle. Understanding the changes brought by both the cancer and the cancer treatment can help patients make the most of this time. Because recurrence is unfortunately a common event in both esophageal and gastric cancers, for many patients this time may be viewed as the eye of the storm, a time to get back to your life and to make plans for the future when the cancer may return.

## EMOTIONAL HEALING

When treatment ends, you may expect life to return to the way it was before you were diagnosed with cancer, but it can take time to recover. Your body will likely have scars. You may not be able to do some things you once did easily. You may think that others see you differently now, or you may view yourself in a different way. One of the hardest adjustments after treatment is not knowing what will happen next. What was once "normal" for you may have changed. There may be changes in the way you look, in the way you eat, in the things you do, and in your relationships with others. Although you may wish to put the cancer behind you, your emotional recovery may be just beginning. Your cancer center checkups may become less frequent, and while on the surface, this is a good thing, going to the hospital or clinic often gives patients a sense of security. Many people describe feeling abandoned and a little frightened when they no longer are in such frequent contact with their doctors and nurses.

You may experience significant anxiety about the cancer coming back. You may be very frustrated if you are unable to just get on with your life as before. You may have trouble relating to your relatives and friends, and they may be unsure how to respond to you. In response to these difficulties, you may wish to develop a wellness plan that includes ways you can address your physical, social, and spiritual needs. If your doctor or a friend suggests that you consider seeing a counselor, try not to be angry or offended. Many patients benefit from seeing a therapist after treatment to assist them in the adjustment of reengaging in their lives both physically and emotionally. Recovering from cancer and cancer treatment can be the same as recovering from a post-traumatic stress disorder. Certainly, cancer and cancer treatment is a major stress. Remember, you are not alone, and what you are experiencing is the norm—not the exception.

## LONG-TERM EFFECTS OF CANCER AND TREATMENT

Both cancer and cancer treatment may lead to many changes in your body. Your doctor has ways to help you deal with many of these changes and can minimize the effects these changes have on your life. Cancer treatment can leave patients with a number of symptoms such as fatigue, loss of appetite, joint pain, peripheral neuropathy, and anemia. Fatigue can linger for a year. Give your body time to heal and adjust.

## PAIN

Some people may have significant pain after treatment, while others have less or none at all. The pain following surgery is usually short term, lasting a matter of weeks. Narcotic pain medicines are usually prescribed, and the pattern of pain and narcotic use following surgery rarely predisposes to tolerance or addiction, so you can be liberal taking the pain medicines. Chronic pain can be more difficult to manage and requires careful discussion and reevaluation with your care team. Initially, pain is managed with anti-inflammatory medications and narcotics. In most cases, doctors will try the milder medicines first. They will then work up to stronger ones if you need them. To keep ongoing pain under control, do not skip doses. Antidepressant medicines may be prescribed to reduce the pain or numbness caused by peripheral neuropathy. Physical therapy can use heat, cold, massage or pressure, and exercise to make you feel better. Acupuncture is a proven method using needles at specific pressure points to reduce pain. Many people have found that practicing deep relaxation such as meditation, yoga, or hypnosis relieves or reduces stress and pain. While going through cancer treatment can be uncomfortable, much of this discomfort will go away when the treatment stops. If it does not, discuss the discomfort with your doctor.

## LIVING WELL AFTER TREATMENT: NOURISHING YOUR BODY, MIND, AND SPIRIT

The key to living well after cancer treatment is taking ownership of your own health. For months, teams of doctors, nurses, and other professionals will be carefully caring for you. Although you are a key player on this team, once these treatments have stopped, you may find yourself more in the driver's seat, as the decisions made do not involve complicated medical techniques or medications. While your doctor is there to support and guide you, this is the time for you to "carry the ball."

### DIET AND NUTRITION

You have just had surgery and many treatments on important parts of your digestive tract; your body is likely to have undergone some changes in gastrointestinal function.

After surgery, you may find that you do not feel as well after eating some foods or after large meals. As mentioned previously, your energy level may be slow to return, in part because of anemia but also because your body may not have the ability to digest food properly and extract the nutritious substances that keep you alert and active.

If you have had a gastrectomy or esophagectomy, your doctor may provide you with dietary guidelines. A postgastrectomy diet is designed to meet the health needs of patients who have had surgery of the upper gastrointestinal tract (see Table 1). It can help slow down the rate at which food travels through the gastrointestinal tract, giving your body more time to digest food and extract needed nutrients.

## ACTIVITY AND MOBILITY

While pain may resolve and your appetite may return in the weeks and months after treatments have stopped, patients often find their energy level takes much longer to fully recover. If you have had chemotherapy, it may take 2–3 months or even a year for your energy to return to its pretreatment level. Cancer treatment often contributes to anemia and changes in nutritional status that can take a while to overcome. Do not overdo it. This is not a time to push yourself too hard. Give your body and your blood a good long chance to recover.

Cancer treatments do not often affect a patient's mobility. As you recover some of your energy, your mobility will remain or return to its level before chemotherapy. Likewise, fatigue may have an effect on sexual activity. Give yourself time to recover, and when your energy level returns, you

**TABLE 1:** POSTGASTRECTOMY DIET (HERE ARE SOME DIETARY
TREATMENT STRATEGIES THAT YOUR DOCTOR MAY RECOMMEND):

- Eat more frequently and eat smaller meals. Eating six small meals a day can help avoid overloading the stomach.

- Avoid drinking liquids with meals. Drink liquids only between meals, such as 30 minutes before a meal or 1 hour after a meal. If you do drink with a meal, keep the amount small (1/2 cup).

- Lie down and put your feet up for at least 15 minutes after every meal. This may slow down the movement of food into your intestines.

- Change your diet to include more fiber and protein.

- Eat more fruit, which can contain both fiber and pectin— substances that help keep carbohydrates around longer to allow for better digestion.

- Avoid or eat fewer simple carbohydrates such as sweets, candy, cookies, cakes, and foods that contain glucose, sucrose, fructose, dextrose, honey, and corn syrup (read the labels). Avoid soft drinks.

- Avoid very acidic foods (tomatoes, oranges, lemons, limes, grapefruit) as they may be hard to digest. Similarly, avoid deep-fried food.

- To make up for some for the nutrients that may be missing in your diet or hard for your GI tract to absorb, take a multivitamin prescribed by your doctor. Important vitamins at this time often include iron, calcium, folate, and vitamin B12 (B12 is sometimes given as a monthly injection).

should soon be back to your pretreatment level of sexual activity. Make sure that you get enough sleep during this recovery period. When you feel up to it, gentle exercise is a good way to help you return to your previous fitness level.

SELF-CARE

In addition to a good diet that follows postgastrectomy guidelines (if you have had a gastrectomy or esophagec-tomy), good sleep, and maybe some gentle activity, there are things you can do to further enhance your health. Complementary medicine techniques such as acupuncture and massage can have wonderful effects on your return to health. Look for licensed practitioners, many of whom have experience supporting cancer patients. Look for ways to help your body cope with stress. Techniques such as deep breathing, yoga, and meditation have proven very effective at helping many people deal with life's stresses. Likewise, avoid habits that may negatively affect your health such as smoking, alcohol, and substance abuse.

## FAITH, RELIGION, OR SPIRITUALITY

Having a serious illness such as cancer can affect your spiritual outlook. For some, their spirituality may get stronger. Others may question their faith or the meaning of life and their role in life. Many say they develop a new focus and live day by day, trying to live each day to its fullest. Through faith, many cancer survivors have been able to find meaning in their lives and make sense of their cancer experience. Often the religious community provides an avenue for patients to connect with others, including some who have shared similar experiences. Religion can provide an outlet for coping and recovering from cancer. Seeking answers and searching for personal meaning in spirituality can offer hope, perspective, and comfort.

## SUPPORT GROUPS

There are many different types of cancer support groups. Support groups offer opportunities to connect with other cancer survivors who have had similar experiences. Support groups can allow for sharing of personal stories. Telling and hearing stories about living with cancer can help you voice your concerns, face problems, or find meaning in what you have been through. You can discover humor and laughter in your cancer experience. When you laugh, your brain releases chemicals that produce pleasure and relax your muscles. Laughter or even a smile can help fight off stress. You can also learn from a support group about ways to handle symptoms and side effects of treatment, or about treatment options and how others have handled situations similar to your own. The support group may be led by a health professional or by a fellow cancer survivor. The Internet can provide access to informal chat groups. However, while these online groups can provide emotional support, they may not always provide correct medical information, and you need to be careful about making any changes based on what you read. Ask your doctor, who knows your cancer and your situation, about any medical advice you receive online.

## SEEING THE WORLD THROUGH DIFFERENT EYES

Following treatment is a good time to step back and reassess your life. What may have seemed important before may be less so now. Consider setting short-term and long-term goals. These goals may be directed at a healthier lifestyle for yourself or at readjusting how or with whom you are spending your time. Find ways to help yourself relax. Spend quiet time at home, or simply get out of the house; this can help you focus on other things besides cancer and the worries it brings. If you have recovered fully from your cancer and treatment, you may wish to consider what you can contribute to the treatment of cancer. You could volunteer at the cancer center where you received your treatment or with an organization such as the American Cancer Society.

This experience has changed you. Life may be more precious and valued than it was before. You have had to face your own mortality and have shared this experience with close family and friends. Use the connections you have made to continue pursuing what is now valuable to you. Make use of this new lease on life.

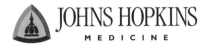

# CHAPTER 8

# MANAGING RISK—WHAT IF MY CANCER COMES BACK?

If gastric or esophageal cancer has been removed and there is no sign of spread to distant organs, then you hope to be cured. Even if there is no sign of spread and the tumor was removed at surgery with negative margins, you may still have cancer cells in your body. Knowing that you could possibly still have cancer is part of what it means to be a cancer survivor. Your doctors will follow you with scheduled visits and tests to look for any sign of cancer recurrence. For these tumors, you have to wait 5 years before you or your doctors can declare you cured. This waiting period is because if cancer of the esophagus or stomach recurs, it usually does so within the first few years; if 5 years have passed with no sign of cancer, the chance of recurrence becomes vanishingly small.

Unfortunately, the majority of patients with gastroesophageal cancer will have cancer recurrence. This can sometimes be hard to understand. When a doctor or patient says cancer "came back" or "recurred," it didn't really come back; rather cancer was present all along, though not detectable. If the cancer has not yet spread beyond the area treated, then removing it by surgery or treating with radiation and chemotherapy has a chance of being curative. If cancer cells have already spread beyond the area of treatment, they will eventually become evident. For cancer in the esophagus or stomach, detecting cancer at any time after treatment is a very bad sign. Unlike many other cancers, esophageal or gastric cancer usually cannot be cured if it recurs.

## MONITORING FOR RECURRENCE

The risk of recurrence is greatest within the first 2 years of the diagnosis. Recurrence can cause symptoms of difficulty swallowing or eating, anemia, or unexplained weight loss. The National Comprehensive Cancer Network (NCCN) guidelines suggest a physical examination every 3 to 6 months for 3 years, and then once a year until the 5-year mark is reached. Both the surgical oncologist and the medical oncologist will usually provide this follow-up care. If there is no evidence of recurrence after 5 years of follow-up, patients can continue to be followed by their primary care doctor or family physician. CT scan can either be followed regularly or based on a patient's health. Eating or swallowing difficulty may prompt an upper endoscopy to evaluate for recurrence. Doctors refer to "local" versus "distant" recurrence. Local recurrence refers to tumor coming back in the same area of the body where it first occurred.

The risk of local recurrence is usually lower in patients who received radiation therapy. Distant recurrence is spread to other organs. When stomach or esophageal cancer recurs in a distant organ, the most common sites are the liver, lungs, and bones. This newly found cancer is not considered "liver cancer," "lung cancer," or "bone cancer," however; it is gastroesophageal cancer cells that have traveled to these organs and established themselves there.

## MANAGEMENT OF RECURRENT GASTROESOPHAGEAL CANCER

For almost all people, recurrence of gastric or esophageal cancer is incurable with the currently available therapies. Further surgery is not likely to be recommended, as it will not increase survival or relieve symptoms. Patients with obstruction of the esophagus and trouble swallowing may be offered endoscopic laser treatment to try to open the esophagus, or placement of a metallic stent to keep a passage open to the stomach. In severe cases, a feeding tube is required to provide nutritional support. Radiation treatment, if not already given to an area, can help with localized pain due to bone involvement or can shrink (but not eliminate) the local tumor. When the cancer recurs distally, the treatment depends on the patient's overall health status and the estimated length of survival. If additional chemotherapy is needed or recommended, the drugs may be different than those used before.

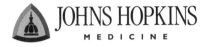

# CHAPTER 9

# My Cancer Isn't Curable— What Now?

## UNDERSTANDING TREATMENT GOALS FOR METASTATIC DISEASE

It can be devastating to hear that your disease has gone beyond your stomach or esophagus and your lymphatic system and has been found in another organ. This changes the treatment plan from one of attempted cure to one of cancer control. The goal of treatment is to try to control the disease and keep your body in harmony with the disease as long as possible while maintaining good quality of life. This effort requires a careful balance. A good quality of life is just as important, if not more so, than focusing on how many weeks, months, or years are left. Living a long time in pain or unable to care for your daily needs and not enjoying your life is not a goal. A shortened time during which you feel pretty good and enjoy friends and family is far better than being miserable for a longer time. If you are experiencing significant pain, tell you doctors and nurses. There are medications and treatments to control pain. Sometimes patients are frightened to report pain or new symptoms, fearing they will be told the prognosis has worsened. The doctors and nurses may not know you are suffering if you don't tell them. There may be specific treatments that can markedly improve or alleviate your pain.

## DECIDING WHEN TO STOP TREATMENT

"When should I stop treatment?" is not an easy question to ask your doctor; nor is it an easy question for him or her to answer. You should have a candid discussion with your doctor about what the stopping point for treatment is. This may require you to meet with your doctor one-on-one without your family. It is often easier to speak frankly when your spouse, son, or daughter is not sitting right beside you. It is, of course, your decision which family members should be present when talking with your treatment team. In general, treatment continues as long as you are responding and your quality of life is being maintained. There is no sense continuing treatment, however, if it is not helping. You will want your doctor to be both open and honest with you. It will be hard for him or her to recommend stopping treatment, just as it is hard for you to hear those words. Physicians are trained to make patients feel better, to heal, to cure, to take pain away, and to reduce suffering. It is difficult to tell a patient that further treatment will not help, but it is important that they say so if and when such a time occurs. Being prepared for such a time is wise. This means asking the doctor how long he or she anticipates being able to hold the cancer back and asking if there are any other treatments that can be offered if your current treatment fails.

You should have your affairs in order and make your wishes about treatment and death known. Most people postpone or avoid doing this, perhaps in part due to denial. Everyone, whether or not they have cancer, will at some point have to put their affairs in order. Life is unpredictable. Your cancer provides you a window into your future and what timeline it holds for you. Take advantage of this knowledge, and make sure you have a will, an advanced directive, your finances in order, and your wishes clearly known to your family.

## HOSPICE/PALLIATIVE CARE

When cancer patients reach the end of their life, there are special medical services available to help them prepare for passing on. Hospice is a philosophy of care that accepts death as the final stage of life. This includes dying with dignity, with pain in control, and having your family's emotional needs met. Your doctor can arrange the referral to hospice, which is often done around the time that the decision is made that treatment is no longer benefiting you.

Hospice care treats the patient rather than the disease. Care is provided for the patient and the family 24 hours a day, 7 days a week. Doctors, nurses, social workers, counselors, home health aides, clergy, therapists, and trained volunteers care for you and offer support based on their areas of expertise. Together, they provide complete palliative care aimed at relieving symptoms and giving social, emotional, and spiritual support. Hospice care can be provided in a specialized hospice facility, in your own home, or in the home of a relative. It's your choice. Most hospice care in the United States is provided in the home, with a family member, or even multiple members serving as the main caregivers. Members of the hospice staff visit regularly to check on you and your family and give needed care and services. Home hospice programs have an on-call nurse who answers phone calls day and night, makes home visits, or sends the appropriate team member if needed between scheduled visits. Medicare-certified hospices provide nursing, pharmacy, and doctor services around the clock.

Hospice care is suitable when you no longer benefit from cancer treatment and are expected to live 6 months or less. Hospice gives you palliative care with treatment to help relieve cancer-related symptoms, but not cure the disease. You, your family, and your doctor decide when hospice care should begin. Sometimes the doctor, patient, or family member will resist hospice because he or she feels it sends a message of hopelessness. This is not true. The hope that hospice brings is the hope of quality living, making the best of each day during the last stages of advanced illness. Quality of the final chapter of your life is most important. Honoring your wishes and spending time as you want to spend it is now the goal. Counseling is provided to family members, and spiritual needs are addressed. This is your time with family and friends; this is your time for reflection and to gain peace.

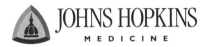

# CHAPTER 10

# CANCER OF THE STOMACH AND ESOPHAGUS IN OLDER ADULTS

*Gary R. Shapiro, MD*

M ost cases of esophageal and gastric cancer occur in patients 65 years of age or older. As we live longer, the number of people with cancers of esophagus and stomach will increase. In the next 25 years, the number of people who are 65 years of age and older will double, and the largest increases in cancer incidence will occur in those older than 80 years of age. This is already the case for gastric cancer, where, despite its declining overall incidence, the number of octogenarians with gastric cancer is growing with each passing year.

Older adults with cancer often have other chronic health problems, and may be taking multiple medications that can affect their cancer treatment plan. Prejudice, misunderstanding, and limited access to clinical trials often prevent older patients from getting the timely cancer treatment that they need.

Older men and woman may not have adequate screening for esophageal and gastric cancers, and when a cancer is found, it is too often ignored or undertreated. As a result, older individuals often have more advanced stage cancer and worse outcomes than younger patients.

## WHY IS THERE MORE CANCER IN OLDER PEOPLE?

The organs in our body are made up of cells. Cells divide and multiply as the body needs them. Cancer develops when cells in a part of the body grow out of control. The body has a number of ways of repairing damaged control mechanisms, but as we get older, these do not work as well. Although our healthier lifestyles have allowed us to avoid death from infection, heart attack and stroke, we may now live long enough for a cancer to develop. People who live longer have increased exposure to cancer-causing agents (carcinogens) in the environment (like tobacco, alcohol, and *Helicobacter pylori* infections). Aging decreases the body's ability to protect us from these carcinogens and to repair cells that are damaged by these and other processes (like gastroesophageal acid reflux, peptic ulcers, and pernicious anemia described in Chapter 1).

## ESOPHAGEAL & GASTRIC CANCERS ARE DIFFERENT IN OLDER PEOPLE

There are two types of esophageal cancer; squamous cell cancer and adenocarcinoma (see Chapter 1). The squamous cell type can occur anywhere in the esophagus and it is related to smoking and drinking large quantities of alcohol. It is on the decline in younger people, but still quite prevalent in older people who grew up in a less health conscious era. Adenocarcinomas of the esophagus occur at the lowest end of the esophagus and are associated with gastroesophageal acid reflux disease. The overwhelming majority of the millions of people who have acid reflux do not get cancer, but those who have changes in the esophagus seen by endoscopy called Barrett's esophagus have a much higher chance and have to be followed closely. Patients with Barrett's esophagus are followed by repeat endoscopy and biopsy. Since older people have more time for exposure to these cancer-causing effects of acid reflux, it is no surprise that the number of people with adenocarcinoma of the esophagus is increasing as people live longer. Risk factors for stomach cancer include gastric polyps, pernicious anemia, prior *H. pylori* infection (the bacteria associated with peptic ulcers), and prior stomach surgery (in which part of the stomach was removed). Stomach cancer is usually adenocarcinoma. There are two types of stomach adenocarcinoma. The intestinal variety of adenocarcinoma of the stomach arises in areas of the stomach affected by chronic atrophic gastritis, and, since it takes years to develop, it is more common in the elderly. This type of stomach cancer has a localized growth pattern, and local resection of the tumor by endoscopy may be adequate treatment. The diffuse type of stomach adenocarcinoma occurs more often in women, tends to occur at younger age, and can spread through the stomach wall. This is often called signet ring type because of a typical appearance of some cancer cells under the microscope.

Multiple areas of cancer in the stomach are more common in the elderly than in their younger counterparts.

## DECISION MAKING: 7 PRACTICAL STEPS

### 1. GET A DIAGNOSIS

No matter how "typical" the signs and symptoms, first impressions are sometimes wrong. That suspicious stomach mass may not be an adenocarcinoma, but a lymphoma that, though malignant, requires relatively simple treatment. It might even be benign. A diagnosis helps you and your family understand what to expect and how to prepare for the future, even if you cannot get curative treatment. Knowing the diagnosis also helps your doctor treat your symptoms better. Many people find "not knowing" very hard, and are relieved when they finally have an explanation for their symptoms. Sometimes a frail patient is obviously dying, and diagnostic studies can be an additional burden. In such cases, it may be quite reasonable to focus on symptom relief (palliation) without knowing the details of the diagnosis.

### 2. KNOW THE CANCER'S STAGE

The cancer's stage defines your prognosis and treatment options. No one can make informed decisions without it. Just as there may be times when the burdens of diagnostic studies may be too great, it may also be appropriate to do without full staging in very frail, dying patient.

As it is in younger patients, stage is determined by the size of the tumor, the presence or absence of cancer in lymph nodes or its spread (metastasis) to other organs. When doctors combine this information with information regarding your cancer's site of origin and tissue type, they can predict what impact, if any, your gastroesophageal cancer is likely to have on your life expectancy and quality of life.

## 3. KNOW YOUR LIFE EXPECTANCY

Anticancer treatment should be considered if you are likely to live long enough to experience symptoms or premature death from gastric or esophageal cancer. If your life expectancy is so short that the cancer will not significantly affect it, there may be no reason to treat your cancer.

However, chronological age (how old you are) should not be the only thing that decides how your cancer should, or should not, be treated. Despite advanced age, people who are relatively well often have a life expectancy that is longer than their life expectancy with esophageal or gastric cancer. The average 70-year-old woman is likely to live another 16 years, and the average 70-year-old man another 12 years. A similar 85-year-old can expect to live an additional 5 to 6 years, and remain independent for most of that time. Even an unhealthy 75-year-old man or woman probably will live 5 to 6 more years—long enough to suffer symptoms and early death from recurrent gastroesophageal cancer.

## 4. UNDERSTAND THE GOALS

**The Goals of Treatment**

It is important to be clear whether the goal of treatment is cure (surgery, chemo-radiation therapy, or all three combined for early, stage gastric or esophageal cancer) or palliation (radiation or chemotherapy for incurable locally advanced or metastatic gastric or esophageal cancer). If the goal is palliation, you need to understand if the treatment plan will extend your life, control your symptoms, or both. How likely is it to achieve these goals, and how long will you enjoy its benefits?

When the goal of treatment is palliation, chemotherapy should never be administered without defined endpoints and timelines. It should be clear to everyone what counts as success, how it will be determined (for example, a symptom controlled or a smaller mass on CT scan), and when. You and your family should understand what your options are at each step, and how likely each is to meet your goals. If this is not clear, ask your doctor to explain it in words that you understand.

### The Goals of the Patient

In addition to the traditional goals of tumor response, increased survival, and symptom control, older cancer patients often have goals related to quality of life. These may include physical and intellectual independence, spending quality time with your family, taking trips, staying out of the hospital, or even economic stability. At times, palliative care or hospice may meet these goals better than active anticancer treatment. In addition to the medical team, older patients often turn to family, friends, and clergy to help guide them.

### 5. DETERMINE IF YOU ARE FIT OR FRAIL

Deciding how to treat cancer in someone who is older requires a thorough understanding of her general health and social situation. Decisions about cancer treatment should never focus on age alone.

### Age is Not a Number

Your actual age (chronological age) has limited influence on how cancer will respond to therapy or its prognosis. Biological and other changes associated with aging are more reliable in estimating an individual's vigor, life expectancy, or the risk of treatment complications. These changes include malnutrition, loss of muscle mass and strength, depression, dementia, falls, social isolation, and the ability to accomplish daily activities such as dressing, bathing, eating, shopping, housekeeping, and managing one's finances or medication.

### Chronic Illnesses

Older cancer patients are likely to have chronic illnesses (comorbidity) that affect their life expectancy; the more that you have, the greater the effect. This effect has very little impact on the behavior of the cancer itself, but studies do show that comorbidity has a major impact on treatment outcome and its side effects.

## 6. BALANCE BENEFITS AND HARMS

Fit older gastric and esophageal cancer patients respond to treatment similarly to their younger counterparts. However, a word of caution is in order. Until recently, few studies included older individuals, and it may not be appropriate to apply these findings to the diverse group of older cancer patients.

The side effects of cancer treatment are never less in the elderly. In addition to the standard side effects, there are significant age-related toxicities to consider. Though most of these are more a function of frailty than chronological age, even the fittest senior cannot avoid the physical effects of aging. In addition to the changes in fat and muscle that you see in the mirror, there are age-related changes in your kidney, liver, and digestive (gastrointestinal) function. These changes affect how your body absorbs and metabolizes anticancer drugs and other medicines. The average senior takes many different medicines (to control, for example, high blood pressure, high cholesterol, osteoporosis, diabetes, arthritis, etc.). This "polypharmacy" can cause undesirable side effects as the many drugs interact with each other and the anticancer medications.

7. GET INVOLVED

Healthcare providers and family members often underestimate the physical and mental abilities of older people and their willingness to face chronic and life-threatening conditions. Studies clearly show that older patients want detailed and easily understood information about potential treatments and alternatives. Patients and families may consider cancer untreatable in the aged, and not understand the possibilities offered by treatment.

While patients with dementia pose a unique challenge, they are frequently capable of participating in goal setting and simple discussions about treatment side effects and logistics. Caring family members and friends are often able to share the patient's life story so that healthcare workers can work with them to make decisions consistent with the patient's values and desires. This of course is no substitute for a well thought out and properly executed Living Will or healthcare proxy.

While it is hard to face the possibility of life-threatening events at any age, it is always better to be prepared and to "put your affairs in order." In addition to estate planning and wills, it is critical that you outline your wishes regarding medical care at the end of life, and make legal provisions for someone to make those decisions if you are unable to make them for yourself.

## TREATING GASTRIC AND ESOPHAGEAL CANCER

### YOU NEED A TEAM

Cancer care changes rapidly, and it is hard for the generalist to keep up to date, so referral to a specialist is essential. The needs of an older cancer patient often extend beyond the doctor's office and the traditional services provided by visiting nurses. These needs may include transportation, nutrition, emotional, financial, physical or spiritual support. When an older woman or man with gastroesophageal cancer is the primary care giver for a frail or ill spouse, grandchildren or other family members, special attention is necessary to provide for their needs as well. Older cancer patients cared for in geriatric oncology programs benefit from multidisciplinary teams of oncologists, geriatricians, psychiatrists, pharmacists, physiatrists, social workers, nurses, clergy, and dieticians, all working together as a team to identify and manage the stressors that can limit effective cancer treatment.

SURGERY

Though gastric and esophageal cancer surgery is often complex, it is the standard of care for most early stage cancers of the stomach and esophagus (see Chapter 3), regardless of age. Like other treatment options, surgery in some older individuals may involve risks related to decreases in body organ function (especially heart and lung), and it is essential that the surgeon and anesthetist work closely with your primary care physician (or a consultant) to fully assess and treat these problems before, during, and after the operation.

As in younger patients, cure rates depend on cancer stage, histology, grade, and the number of lymph nodes affected by the cancer. Surgery is as effective in elderly patients as in younger patients, but it does have a somewhat higher rate of complications in older individuals (especially those over 80) who have other medical problems (comorbidities). Chemo-radiation therapy for gastric cancer is only palliative, and it is no substitute for potentially curable surgery in early stage resectable gastric cancer. On the other hand, cure may be possible when definitive chemo-radiation therapy (see page 39) is used to treat some stages of esophageal cancer that have not spread to distant sites. This type of aggressive therapy is not without risk, and older people who are too frail to undergo curative surgery may also be too frail to get curative chemo-radiation therapy for their esophageal cancer. Therefore, it is essential that you weigh all of the risks and benefits with your multidisciplinary care team. Minimally invasive (laparoscopic) surgery is another option that you may wish to discuss with your doctors (see page 36).

Endoscopic mucosal resection (EMR) is a low risk, easily tolerated, effective alternative to esophagectomy or gastrectomy in both fit and frail individuals whose cancer is confined to the superficial mucosal lining (stage T1a) of the esophagus or stomach. Patients with problems swallowing due to locally advanced or recurrent esophageal cancer, or those too frail to tolerate definitive local therapy (surgery or radiation therapy with or without chemotherapy), often get relief from an esophageal stent placed through an endoscope.

## RADIATION THERAPY

In the absence of concurrent chemotherapy, the effects of radiation therapy are limited. Although it is rarely curative, it often provides local palliation, and may even prolong life, in esophageal cancer patients who are unfit for surgery and unable to tolerate chemotherapy. Radiation therapy also provides excellent symptom relief in metastatic and other incurable situations. It is particularly effective in treating pain caused by stomach and esophageal cancer metastases to the bone. In these situations, a short course of radiation therapy often allows patients with advanced cancer to lower (or even eliminate) their dose of narcotic pain relievers. Although these medicines do an excellent job of controlling pain, they often cause confusion, falls, and constipation in older patients. Thus, even hospice patients suffering from localized metastatic bone pain should consider the option of palliative radiation therapy.

Sores (mucositis) and dryness in the mouth and esophagus caused by radiation therapy can be more problematic in older patients who are already at risk for dehydration and malnutrition, but dehydration, weight loss, and electrolyte disturbances can be avoided with carefully monitoring and early treatment. Regular, meticulous inspection of the mouth and prompt treatment to control pain and infection is essential. Feeding tubes help patients receiving radiation therapy (and chemotherapy) get adequate fluid and nutritional support.

The fatigue that usually accompanies radiation therapy can be quite profound in the elderly, even in those who are fit. Often the logistical details (like daily travel to the hospital for a 6–8 week course of treatment) are the hardest for older people. It is important that you discuss these potential problems with your family and social worker, prior to starting radiation therapy.

CHEMOTHERAPY

Non-frail older cancer patients respond to chemotherapy (see Chapter 3) similarly to their younger counterparts. Reducing the dose of chemotherapy (or radiation therapy) based purely on chronological age may seriously affect the effectiveness of treatment. Managing chemotherapy-associated toxicity with appropriate supportive care (like the early placement of feeding tubes) is crucial in the elderly population to give them the best chance of cure and survival, or to provide the best palliation.

In younger patients with stomach cancer, all but the earliest T1 lesions generally get postoperative adjuvant chemoradiation therapy to decrease their risk of cancer recurrence. Sometimes neoadjuvant chemotherapy is recommended before potentially curative surgery for both gastric and esophageal cancer. Only the most robust seniors are able to tolerate this type of intensive multimodality (chemotherapy, radiation therapy, and surgery) therapy, and it is essential that you weigh the burdens and benefits of these aggressive approaches carefully. The additional benefit may only be marginal, and less aggressive approaches (surgery for gastric cancer and esophageal cancer, or definitive chemo-radiation therapy for esophageal cancer) may be more appropriate.

Platinol (cisplatin) is often used in combination chemotherapy regimens, especially when treating esophageal cancer (with or without radiation). Although it is a highly effective agent, the benefit is not without its down side. Older patients have a higher rate of mouth sores (mucositis), diarrhea, thrombocytopenia (low platelet blood count that can cause bleeding), and kidney (nephrotoxicity) side effects. Severe side effects are more common in Platinol-based chemotherapy programs than those that use other drugs.

Though the side effects of cancer treatment are never less burdensome in the elderly, they can be managed by oncologists, especially geriatric oncologists, who work in teams with others who specialize in the care of the elderly. With appropriate care, healthy older patients do just as well with chemotherapy as younger patients. Advances in supportive care (antinausea medicines and blood cell growth factors) have significantly decreased the side effects of chemotherapy, and improved safety and the quality of life of individuals with stomach and esophageal cancer. Nonetheless, there is risk, especially if the patient is frail. The presence of severe comorbidities, age-related frailty or underlying severe psychosocial problems may be obstacles for highly intensive treatment plans. Such patients may benefit from less complicated or potentially less toxic treatment plans.

## COMMON TREATMENT COMPLICATIONS IN THE ELDERLY

Anemia (low red blood cell count) is common in the elderly, especially the frail elderly. It decreases the effectiveness of chemotherapy, and often causes fatigue, falls, cognitive decline (for example, dementia, disorientation, or confusion), and heart problems. Therefore, it is essential that anemia be recognized and corrected with red blood cell transfusions or the appropriate use of erythropoiesis-stimulating agents like Procrit or Epogen (epoetin) or Aranesp (darbepoetin).

Myelosuppression (low white blood cell count) is also common in older patients getting chemotherapy or radiation therapy. Older patients with myelosuppression develop life-threatening infections more often than younger patients, and they may need to be treated in the hospital for many days. The liberal use of G-CSF, Neupogen, Neulasta (granulopoietic growth factors) decreases the risk of infection, and makes it possible for older women to receive full doses of potentially curable adjuvant chemotherapy.

Mucositis (mouth sores) and diarrhea can cause severe dehydration in older patients who often are already dehydrated due to inadequate fluid intake and diuretics (water pills for high blood pressure or heart failure). Careful monitoring and the liberal use of antidiarrheal agents (Imodium) and oral and intravenous fluids are essential components of the management of older cancer patients, especially those receiving radiation or Adrucil, or both.

Xerostomia (dry mouth) and esophagitis may also contribute to dehydration and malnutrition in older esophageal cancer patients. Older patients occasionally have a harder time adapting to this, and other functional disabilities that follow operative and nonoperative treatments, in particular the swallowing problems (dysphagia) that can result from radiation therapy. Many older patients go to nursing homes for several weeks after treatment, and often do not get adequate rehabilitation and swallowing therapy.

Kidney function declines as we age. Some of the medicines that older patients take to treat both their cancer (for example, Platinol, Paraplatin [carboplatin], Bayer, Aleve and Tylenol [NSAIDs]) and noncancer related problems might make this worse. The dehydration that often accompanies cancer and its treatment can put additional stress on the kidneys. Fortunately, it is often possible to minimize these effects by carefully selecting and dosing appropriate drugs, managing "polypharmacy," and preventing dehydration.

Neurotoxicity & Cognitive Effects ("chemo-brain") can be profoundly debilitating in patients who are already cognitively impaired (demented, disoriented, confused, etc.). Elderly patients with a history of falling, hearing loss, or peripheral neuropathy (nerve damage from, for example, diabetes) have decreased energy, and are highly vulnerable to neurotoxic chemotherapy like the taxanes or platinum compounds. Many of the medicines used to control nausea (antiemetics) or decrease the side effects of certain chemotherapeutic agents are also potential neurotoxins. These include Decadron (dexamethasone) (psychosis and agitation), Zantac (ranitidine) (agitation), Benadryl (diphenhydramine), and some of the antiemetics (sedation).

Fatigue is a near universal complaint of older cancer patients. It is particularly a problem for those who are socially isolated or depend upon others to help them with activities of daily living. It is not necessarily related to depression, but can be. Depression is quite common in the elderly. In contrast to younger patients who often respond to a cancer diagnosis with anxiety, depression is the more common disorder in older cancer patients. With proper support and medical attention, many of these patients can safely receive anticancer treatment.

Heart problems increase with age, and it is no surprise that older cancers patients have an increased risk of cardiac complications from intensive surgery, radiation and chemotherapy. Patients treated with Platinol chemotherapy require large amounts of intravenous fluid hydration. This can cause congestive heart failure in patients with heart problems; they need careful monitoring. Atherosclerosis (blood vessel damage from hardening of the arteries) may increase the chances or local radiation therapy toxicity.

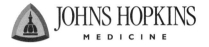

# CHAPTER 11

# TRUSTED RESOURCES—FINDING ADDITIONAL INFORMATION ABOUT CANCER OF THE STOMACH AND ESOPHAGUS AND THEIR TREATMENT

---

For those wanting more information about gastric and esophageal cancer, there is a wealth of educational material and resources available. The following list offers credible and useful organizations and websites that can assist you further.

## American Cancer Society

> (800) ACS-2345
> http://www.cancer.org

This national nonprofit organization provides free educational materials and offers a hotline to address questions of patients and family members dealing with all types of cancer. The American Cancer Society can also provide support services, such as free transportation to chemotherapy treatments for patients without financial means. Additionally, the national office can connect you with their local branch in your geographic region.

## Cancer.Net

> (888) 651-3038
> http://www.cancer.net/portal/site/patient
> Email: cancernet@asco.org

This is the official patient information website of the American Society of Clinical Oncology (ASCO). It provides information about gastrointestinal and other cancers.

## National Cancer Institute (NCI)

> (800) 4-CANCER (NCI's cancer information service)
> http://www.cancer.gov

This organization provides information about all types of cancer, including excellent information about cancer of the esophagus and stomach and how they are treated. You can request free information by calling the toll-free number.

**National Comprehensive Cancer Network (NCCN)**
http://www.nccn.org/

The NCCN is an alliance of 21 of the world's leading cancer centers that are working together to develop treatment guidelines for most cancers, and are dedicated to research that improves the quality, effectiveness, and efficiency of cancer care. NCCN offers a number of programs to help you and your family make informed decisions about your cancer care.

## WHERE CAN I GET HELP WITH FINANCIAL OR LEGAL CONCERNS?

Accompanying any serious illness are questions and concerns related to expenses incurred as a result of treatment, health insurance questions that can be overwhelming to try to understand or resolve, and sometimes even legal questions related to employment or financial matters. The following resources can help you address these concerns.

**CancerCare, Inc.**
(212) 712-8400
(800) 813-HOPE
http://www.cancercare.org
Email: info@cancercare.org

CancerCare is a national nonprofit organization that provides free, professional assistance to people with any type of cancer and to their families. This organization offers education, one-on-one counseling, financial assistance for non-medical expenses, and referrals to community services.

**National Coalition for Cancer Survivorship**

(301) 650-9127
(877) NCSS-YES (to order the Cancer Survival
Toolbox)
http://www.canceradvocacy.org
Email: info@canceradvocacy.org

This network of independent groups and individuals provides information and resources about cancer support,
advocacy, and quality-of-life issues and also helps cancer
patients deal with insurance issues, job discrimination issues, or other related legal matters.

**Patient Advocate Foundation**

(800) 532-5274
http://www.patientadvocate.org
Email: help@patientadvocate.org

This organization provides educational information about
managed care and insurance issues and legal counseling
on debt intervention, job discrimination issues, and insurance denials of coverage.

**ABOUT JOHNS HOPKINS MEDICINE**

Johns Hopkins Medicine unites physicians and scientists
of the Johns Hopkins University School of Medicine with
the organizations, health professionals, and facilities of the
Johns Hopkins Health System. This includes facilities at
the Johns Hopkins Hospital and the Johns Hopkins Bayview Medical Center, in addition to other treatment locations. The mission of Johns Hopkins Medicine is to improve
the health of the community and the world by setting the

standard of excellence in medical education, research, and clinical care. Diverse and inclusive, Johns Hopkins Medicine has provided international leadership in the education of physicians and medical scientists in biomedical research and in the application of medical knowledge to sustain health since the Johns Hopkins Hospital opened in 1889.

### The Johns Hopkins Cancer Surgery Second Opinion Program
(410) 550-HOPE
http://www.hopkinsbayview.org/secondopinion

This program in the Department of Surgery offers those recently diagnosed with esophageal or gastric cancer (as well as other gastrointestinal, breast, or lung cancer) the ability to consult with some of the leading experts in cancer surgery.

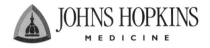

# INFORMATION ABOUT
# JOHNS HOPKINS

---

**The Johns Hopkins Cancer Surgery Second Opinion
Program**

(410) 550-HOPE

http://www.hopkinsbayview.org/secondopinion

This program in the Department of Surgery offers those recently diagnosed with esophageal or gastric cancer (as well as other gastrointestinal, breast, or lung cancers) the ability to consult with some of the leading experts in cancer surgery.

**The Sidney Kimmel Comprehensive Cancer Center at
Johns Hopkins**

http://www.hopkinskimmelcancercenter.org

Since its inception in 1973, the Sidney Kimmel Comprehensive Cancer Center at Johns Hopkins has been dedicated to better understanding human cancers and finding more effective treatments. One of only forty cancer centers in the country designated by the National Cancer Institute (http://www.cancer.gov) as a Comprehensive Cancer Center, the Johns Hopkins Kimmel Comprehensive Cancer Center has active programs in clinical research, laboratory research, education, community outreach, and prevention and control.

### Johns Hopkins Medicine

http://www.hopkinsmedicine.org

Johns Hopkins Medicine unites physicians and scientists of the Johns Hopkins University School of Medicine with the organizations, health professionals, and facilities of the Johns Hopkins Health System. This includes facilities at the Johns Hopkins Hospital and the Johns Hopkins Bayview Medical Center, in addition to other treatment locations. The mission of Johns Hopkins Medicine is to improve the health of the community and the world by setting the standard of excellence in medical education, research, and clinical care. Diverse and inclusive, Johns Hopkins Medicine has provided international leadership in the education of physicians and medical scientists in biomedical research and in the application of medical knowledge to sustain health since the Johns Hopkins Hospital opened in 1889.

# FURTHER READING

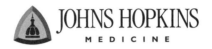

# FURTHER READING

*100 Questions & Answers About Esophageal Cancer, Second Edition,* Pamela K. Ginex, EdD, RN, OCN, Maureen Jingeleski, RN, BSN, Bart L. Frazzitta, and Manjit S. Bains, MD, Jones & Bartlett Learning, 2010.

*100 Questions & Answers About Gastric Cancer,* Manish A. Shah, MD, Natasha A. Pinheiro, RN, BSN, Brinda Shawh, RPh, Jones & Bartlett Learning, 2008.

*100 Questions & Answers About Gastroesophageal Reflux Disease (GERD): A Lahey Clinic Guide,* David L. Burns, MD, CNSP, Neeral L. Shah, MD, Jones & Bartlett Learning, 2007.

*100 Questions & Answers About Gastrointestinal Stromal Tumor (GIST),* Ronald DeMatteo, MD, Marina Symcox, PhD, Jones & Bartlett Learning, 2008.

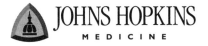

# GLOSSARY

---

**Adenocarcinoma:** Cancer of the tissue-lining cells with gland formation.

**Adjuvant therapy:** Treatment (usually chemotherapy or radiation) given after the primary treatment to increase the chance of cure, and treatment to try to prevent the cancer from recurring.

**Antiemetics:** Medicines to counteract nausea.

**Barrett's esophagus:** A change in the lining cells of the distal esophagus.

**Biopsy:** A procedure in which cells are collected for microscopic examination.

**Bone scan:** An X-ray that evaluates the bones for metastases.

**Brachytherapy:** A form of internal radiation therapy.

**Cancer:** Malignant cells; an invasive tumor.

**Carcinogen:** A substance that may cause cancer.

**Carcinoma in situ:** Early cancer changes that are noninvasive; also called high-grade dysplasia or stage 0 cancer.

**Carcinomas:** Cancers that form from the surface cells of tissue including the lining of the esophagus and stomach.

**Cells:** Basic elements of tissue containing a nucleus and the surrounding substance called cytoplasm.

**Chemo brain:** Reduced cognitive function as a side effect of chemotherapy.

**Chemotherapy:** The use of chemical agents (drugs) to systemically treat cancer.

**Chest tube:** A drainage tube surgically placed in the chest to empty accumulated fluid.

**Clinical trial:** A study of a drug or treatment regimen with a large group of people testing the treatment.

**Comorbidity:** A disease or disorder someone already had unrelated to cancer. Examples include diabetes or heart disease.

**Complementary therapy:** Medicines, herbs, or treatments used in conjunction with standard therapies.

**CT scan or CAT scan:** Abbreviation for computed tomography scanning; an imaging technique that uses X-rays to view the internal body structures.

**Drain:** A small tube inserted into a wound or cavity to collect fluid.

**Dysplasia:** Early changes in cells that can lead toward cancer; high grade dysplasia is also called carcinoma in situ.

**EGD:** Abbreviation for esophagogastroduodenoscopy; the use of a lighted scope inserted through the mouth to examine the esophagus, stomach, and duodenum; also called an upper endoscopy.

**Endoscopic ultrasound:** An ultrasound probe advanced on an endoscope to examine the depth of tumors and look for surrounding lymph nodes.

**Endoscopy:** The use of a flexible scope to evaluate the intestinal tract.

**Esophagectomy:** Surgical removal of the esophagus.

**Esophagogastric:** Related to either the esophagus or the stomach.

**Field:** The treatment site.

**5-Fluorouracil (5-FU) (Adrucil):** Chemotherapy agent used in gastric and esophageal cancer.

**Gastrectomy:** Surgical removal of the stomach.

**Gastric:** Related to the stomach.

**G-tube:** A feeding tube placed in the stomach.

**Incidence:** The number of times a disease occurs within a population.

**Informed consent:** The patient's decision to undertake a particular treatment after having been advised of all available treatment options.

**Invasive cancer:** Cancer that breaks through normal tissue boundaries and invades deeper or surrounding areas.

**J-tube:** A feeding tube placed in the small intestine (jejunum).

**Living will:** A document that outlines what care a person wants in the event he or she becomes unable to communicate due to heavy sedation, unresponsiveness, or coma. May also be referred to as an advanced directive.

**Lymph:** Fluid carried through the body by the lymphatic system; composed primarily of white blood cells and diluted plasma.

**Lymphadenectomy:** Surgical removal of lymph nodes from an area of the body.

**Lymph nodes:** Tissues in the lymphatic system that filter the lymph.

**Lymphoma:** A cancer of the lymphatic cells.

**Malignant:** Cancerous cells or tissue.

**Metastasis:** The spread of cancer cells to other sites.

**Mortality:** The calculation of death rates due to a specific disease within a population.

**MRI:** Abbreviation for magnetic resonance imaging; uses magnetic signals rather than x-rays to provide views of the internal body structures.

**Mutation:** Alteration in the DNA of the cells.

**Neoadjuvant therapy:** The use of chemotherapy or chemotherapy plus radiation before surgery.

**Neutropenia:** A condition of abnormally low levels of white blood cells.

**Noninvasive cancer:** Cancer changes in cells confined to the lining of the tissue with no invasion or spread.

**Oncologist:** A cancer specialist.

**Palliative care:** Care to relieve symptoms of cancer and to preserve quality of life for as long as possible without seeking to cure cancer.

**Pathologist:** A specialist trained to distinguish normal from abnormal cells under the microscope.

**PET scan:** Abbreviation for positron emission tomography scan; an imaging technique to look for rapidly growing or active cells.

**Placebo:** A pill with no medicine (such as a sugar pill); its effects are compared to the effects of a medicine to determine if the medicine's value may be psychological.

**Primary care doctor:** Regular medical physician or family doctor.

**Prognosis:** An estimate of the likely outcome of an illness.

**Protocol:** The plan for how a treatment is given.

**Radiation oncologist:** A cancer specialist who uses radiation therapy to treat cancer.

**Radiation therapy:** Use of high-energy X-rays to treat cancer and shrink tumors.

**Red blood cells (RBCs):** Cells in the body whose primary function is to carry oxygen to tissue.

**Risk factors:** Any factors that contribute to an increased probability of getting cancer.

**Squamous cell carcinoma:** A specific type of cancer of the surface cells (such as squamous cell carcinoma of the esophagus).

**Stage:** A numeric ranking of cancer progression.

**Surgical oncologist:** A surgical specialist trained in the surgical removal of cancerous tumors.

**Systemic therapy:** A treatment that affects the whole body.

**Targeted therapy:** Treatment that targets specific molecules involved in carcinogenesis or tumor growth.

**TPN:** Abbreviation for total parenteral nutrition; the administration of intravenous nutrition containing protein, carbohydrates, fats, and essential minerals.

**Tumor:** A mass or lump of tissue.

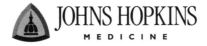